Quest for excellence
in medical education

Quest
for excellence
in medical
education

A personal survey

SIR GEORGE PICKERING

Published for the
Nuffield Provincial Hospitals Trust
by the Oxford University Press

Published for the
Nuffield Provincial Hospitals Trust
3 Prince Albert Road, London NW1 7SP
by Oxford University Press,
Walton Street, Oxford OX2 6DP

Oxford London Glasgow
New York Toronto Melbourne Wellington
Ibadan Nairobi Dar es Salaam Lusaka Cape Town
Kuala Lumpur Singapore Jakarta Hong Kong Tokyo
Delhi Bombay Calcutta Madras Karachi

ISBN 0 19 721399 5

Designed by Bernard Crossland
Printed and bound in Great Britain by
Hazell Watson & Viney Ltd, Aylesbury

Contents

Acknowledgements   vii

1. Introduction   1

The outstanding issues, 2. Undergraduate, graduate, and continuing education, 5. The Medical Acts and their implications, 7.

2. The regulation of medical education   10

The Goodenough Report, 10. The Todd Report, 12. Postgraduate education, 12. Undergraduate education, 13. General Medical Council, 14.

3. Postgraduate (graduate) and continuing education   17

Organization, 18. Pre-registration house appointments, 18. Registrar and senior registrar appointments, 19. The inspection and recognition of training posts, 20. Enrolment of trainees, 21. Assessment of fitness, 21. Examinations, 21. Certification, 22. Formal teaching during training, 22. Career guidance, 23. General comments on graduate education, 24. Advantages, 24. Defects, 24. Use of language, 24. Concentration on examinations, 25. Lack of time, 25. Distance, 25. The huge expense in terms of time and money involved in approving training posts, 25. Rigidity of training, 26. Vocational training for general practice, 27. Postgraduate medical centres, 29. Continuing education, 33. Postgraduate medical education in Scotland, 34.

4. Undergraduate education   36

Quality of students, 37. Size of school, 38. Teaching hospital or district general hospital?, 39. The curriculum, 41. Planning the curriculum, 42. Objectives, 42. General intention, 43. Scientific method, 43. Professional standards, 43. Human biology, 43. Clinical knowledge, 43. Environment and health, 43. Continuing education, 43. Integration, 43. Systems courses and topic teaching, 44. Range of today's curricula, 46. Covering the ground, 47. Present curricula, 47. The role of apprenticeship, 49. Continuous assessment, 50. Reactions to the present curriculum, 53. The remedies, 57. Education in depth, 57. Active and passive learning, 58. The attitude of mind of the teachers, 59. The lecture, 60. The seminar, 60. The ward-round, 60. The out-patients' clinic, 60. The presentation of the patient, 61. Asking individual students to prepare a controversial subject, 61. Training the teacher, 61. Behavioural studies, community medicine, and general practice, 62.

5. Examinations 64

6. The special case of London 71
   Postgraduate education, 71. Undergraduate education, 72.

7. Conclusions 77
   Graduate or postgraduate education for the specialties, 77.
   Undergraduate education, 78. Final comments, 81.

APPENDICES

 I Institutions visited in the course of preparing this
   report 84

II Programme for the month of February for the
   Postgraduate Medical Institute, Stoke on Trent 86

III Report on the Southampton Medical School 88

IV From the Science Masters' Association Report 93

 V Surgery paper from Oxford University, June 1965 99

   References 101

Acknowledgements

I would like to express my gratitude to the Nuffield Provincial Hospitals Trust for their generosity in making this survey possible and for the helpful attitude of their officers. Working with them has been, as always, a pleasure. The Report was carefully criticized in draft by the late Lord Cohen, Professor Archie Duncan, Mr John Potter, and Professor Geoffrey Rose whose criticisms have been gratefully incorporated. I am deeply grateful to Sir Robert Hunter, the Vice-Chancellor of Birmingham University, who enlisted the co-operation and support of the Universities through the Vice-Chancellor's and Principal's Committee. The individual visits were arranged by Miss Gwen Bradfield to whose tact and patience the smooth execution of the survey owes much. My wife accompanied me on as many of these visits as her health permitted. She kept splendid notes and was invaluable in improving and clarifying my English. Finally I owe an especial debt to my secretary, Mrs Patricia Ayling, who kept all the records and typed with great precision the various editions of the Report.

1

Introduction

The Nuffield Provincial Hospitals Trust organized a Conference at Christ Church, Oxford, in 1961 on the subject of postgraduate medical education (1). This was attended by leaders drawn from the university world, the Royal Colleges, and the chief officials of the Ministry of Health. The Conference aroused an intense interest in postgraduate medical education and led to the establishment of postgraduate medical centres at district hospitals throughout England and Wales. These were initially financed by the Trust but afterwards by the Ministry of Health, later the Department of Health and Social Security. In 1973 the Trust organized another Conference at Pembroke College, Oxford (2). As a result, this survey of medical education was commissioned to include undergraduate, postgraduate, and continuing medical education within the framework of the National Health Service.

Through the co-operation of the Committee of Vice-Chancellors and Principals, thirteen medical schools were visited as well as those Royal Colleges and Faculties situated in London (Appendix I). The report is based on these visits and the helpful and critical suggestions of many other leaders of medical thought with whom we discussed the problems. I am particularly grateful to the junior members of staff and students who have spoken so freely of the good and bad aspects of medical education as they have known it and now know it in this country. When I was younger I formed the opinion that nobody was in a better position to comment critically and constructively on education than those who had recently been subjected to it. I have never had any reason to alter this view.

Undergraduate medical education has been the subject of numerous enquiries and reports. The General Medical Council has commissioned a factual survey (3), which is contemporary with this report; although the Goodenough Committee (4) and the Royal Commission (5) devoted their attention to the whole of medical education, postgraduate education was then in its infancy. Now the situation is transformed. Postgraduate education has developed mightily and is a reality which has to be synthesized with that in the undergraduate period. This report, then, is an attempt to look at medical education as a whole and to see the respective roles and purposes of undergraduate, graduate and continuing education and the outstanding needs of each. This is important if the best use is to be made of the splendid young men and women who are now flocking to our medical schools.

Throughout this report I am conscious of the fact that no method has yet been devised to test whether one form of education is superior to another. All assessments are in the nature of value judgements and this is no exception. Others, faced with similar evidence, might have come to different conclusions. In defence of what is written here I can say that it is in essence a distillate of the views of the eager young men and women who have talked to us. For my part, I have been passionately interested in helping the young to develop their curiosity, skills, and critical faculties since I first began as a schoolmaster fifty-one years ago.

Although the value of any particular change in education is impossible to assess objectively and quantitatively, educators have to make the attempt. It may be suggested that the value of medical education can be assessed by:

1. The performance of its graduates in their chosen tasks as general practitioners, specialist physicians or surgeons, medical administrators or research workers.

2. Their liveliness of mind as revealed by interest, originality, and critical ability.

3. Their knowledge.

4. Their ability to communicate facts and ideas accurately and economically to others; in other words, their mastery of written and spoken language (in this case English).

It would be my view that competence and progress should be judged by tests to assess these qualities.

The outstanding issues

Medical education presents a number of objectives which are in conflict. One that runs throughout is the conflict between training the mind as an instrument of precision and enquiry, and training the individual to react quickly and appropriately to specified issues. The first is a function common to all education. It should produce a permanently heightened awareness and capacity for solving problems and arriving at a sound judgement of issues, new or old. The second is a more transient acquisition, for, as practice changes, what may have been an appropriate reaction yesterday becomes inappropriate today and may be less so tomorrow. Because of the Medical Acts and the responsibility of the General Medical Council and licensing bodies to produce people qualified to practise medicine, surgery, and midwifery, the second objective has often taken precedence over the first. It has long been apparent to thoughtful educators that these two objectives should be separated, to some extent at least, in emphasis and time. This has now been achieved or begun to be achieved. The development of graduate and continuing education is specifically designed for doing things, whether it be practice, administration, or research. The undergraduate period is in this way freed for its proper purpose—the training of the mind. This is a matter of no small moment. Today, as never before in Britain, young men and women prefer the career of medicine to all others (6). Those coming into medicine are a highly selected cohort of great ability and great enthusiasm. This survey has revealed that they tend to be disappointed, partly by the low intellectual content of the undergraduate period and the way in which it tends to mould them into a uniform pattern, and partly by the growing inflexibility of the graduate period and the bureaucratic control of the National Health Service. Frustration has been an important cause of emigration in the past, is so in the present and will be in the future. It is therefore of the greatest importance that these faults in our educational system should be recognized and remedied urgently.

The second conflict is an extension of the first. It is the conflict between the needs of the service and the needs of education. This applies particularly to the graduate period. Although the student learns best by doing, and when, in the undergraduate clinical period, he is a member of the team that investigates and advises the sick patient, his responsibilities in this direction are vicarious. In the graduate period, however, he is actually responsible, though that responsibility is limited. The demands made by practice are often so heavy that the graduate student finds too little time for educational purposes. Nor, indeed, are the needs of education the first priority for the average student. At long last he is doing what he wanted—caring for patients. Moreover, the last five years has seen the growth of the trades union mentality, the concept of the forty-hour week and overtime payments. The average graduate occupying a junior hospital post, which is an integral part of his training, tends to regard it as primarily a service post because that brings money while the benefits of education are less tangible and less immediate. The same conflict is experienced by teachers who hold appointments in the NHS rather than a university. There is an increasing tendency to regard service as having priority over teaching, an attitude which is certainly not discouraged by the DHSS.

The task of medical education is to train future doctors. This simple statement conceals several complex issues.

First, there is not just one kind of doctor. His role in the community may range from family doctor through every variety of specialist to community physician, administrator, and research worker.

Second, medical knowledge is expanding and the world is changing. The doctor's task tomorrow may be, and probably will be, very different from that of today.

Third, he does not work *in vacuo*. He has to take his place and solve his problems in the context of the university world at one extreme and that of the NHS at the other. The structure, attitude, and finances of these bodies may play a decisive role.

Finally, the doctor's task is to help his patients to live the fullest lives possible. The doctor himself must therefore have an understanding of the society in which he lives and of the part played in it by government, business, educational, charitable, and other bodies. He must know where to seek help for his patients and how to work with nurses, social workers, and other so-called paramedical professions.

This account of the work of the future doctor makes it plain at the outset that a narrow education or training is not the best preparation for his life's work. What he needs above all is a trained mind. However, it would be a mistake to suppose that the subject matter by which his mind is trained is irrelevant. Any competent craftsman, artist, scientist or any specialist worker must be familiar with his material. In the case of the doctor, his material is man, his mind, his body and his place in society.

The role of the subject matter in training the mind was never better expressed than by the Cambridge University Committee on Education and Business (7) of which Sir Frederick Bartlett, the great psychologist, was a member :

> The view that a university course should not be closely related to a man's ultimate career, but should be a general education in non-vocational subjects, is open to various interpretations. If it is meant that a university course should not consist merely of specific instruction designed to earn one's living, then no objection can be taken to it. If on the other hand the statement is interpreted to mean that a man is best prepared for life by reading subjects wholly unconnected with his career, then a good many objections can be taken to it. Such an interpretation depends ultimately on the assumption that habits of thought are transferable from one subject to another, but there is nothing in experimental psychology to suggest that such transfer will take place automatically.
>
> Any subject can be used as a means of training and developing the intelligence, and when intelligence has been developed by exercise it will be a better instrument for studying other subjects. This, however, is not the same as saying that the clarity of thought attained in one subject is directly transferable to another. In order to secure clarity the ideas involved must be easily manipulated and an early acquaintance with these ideas is a great aid to proficiency. Further, if the subject is one for which the student has special interest, he will more readily advance by using his innate ability unchecked by lack of interest in the subject matter. Perhaps one of the most useful conclusions of experimental psychology has been to stress the importance of developing intelligence in conjunction with special aptitudes and interests and this should be taken into account when considering the desirability of courses for university men going into business.

Undergraduate, graduate, and continuing education

Medical education terminated on graduation for many doctors until the application of the Medical Act of 1953 which required

the satisfactory completion of a year's house jobs in hospital
before full registration. Since then, undergraduate education has
been increasingly supplemented by graduate and continuing education. Undergraduate education should be designed to train the
basic doctor. It would seem obvious that undergraduate education
should have as its principal aim the training of the student's mind
so that he knows how to learn, that he has acquired the basic
discipline of scholarship and the habit of self-education. My
survey has revealed that this is far from the case. Indeed, in many
schools these attitudes and habits are encouraged very seldom or
not at all. In many schools the student who graduates has had
little or no training in how to express himself lucidly and grammatically in speech or writing. He has not the habit of working
in the library, nor has he the habit of asking questions and gath-
ering material so that those questions can be answered. Indeed,
literacy and scholarship are on the decline in our medical schools.
This is by far the most important part of my report.

Graduate education is designed to provide the specialized
knowledge and skills necessary for general practice, specialties
practice, medical administration, and medical research. Continuing education is designed to keep the doctor *au fait* with expanding knowledge and changing practice : it keeps him up to date.

The roles of undergraduate, graduate, and continuing education
are clear enough. But they were not always so. The difficulty
arises from the Medical Acts 1858–1958 requiring the General
Medical Council to ensure that the schools produce doctors competent to practise medicine, surgery, and midwifery. As the only
obligatory education was that ending on graduation or obtaining
the diploma of a licensing body, the undergraduate curriculum
attempted to ensure that this provision was met. In fact it never
was realistic and never could be, as will be discussed in the next
section. The increasing provision of a graduate education which
has as its specific purpose the training of graduates to practise in
that specialty, including general practice, is liberating the undergraduate curriculum for its proper purpose. The last loophole
allowing an improperly trained doctor to practise medicine is
being closed. The National Health Service (Vocational Training)
Act of 1978 (8) is designed to end this by requiring a Health
Authority only to include in its list of medical practitioners undertaking to provide general medical services those who are

'suitably experienced'. It is hoped that this Act will come into full operation in 1980.

By the time those entering medical schools today have completed their medical education and become registered medical practitioners, it seems justifiable to assume that all practitioners of medicine should have had suitable graduate experience.

The considerations just outlined prompted me to ask the regional postgraduate committees and specialty advisers in the centres I was about to visit whether their staff could undertake to teach graduates in their region all the special knowledge and skills needed for specialist practice. In general they agreed that they could, though there remain certain practical difficulties which will be discussed in the main body of the report. They also agreed with the important prerequisite that the student had learned how to learn, and that this was the most important objective of the undergraduate period.

The Medical Acts and their implications

The Annual Report of the General Medical Council for 1975 (9) says

> The present Council's powers do not effectively extend beyond the undergraduate curriculum which should (under the present Medical Acts and in language dating from 1886) 'sufficiently guarantee the possession of the requisite knowledge and skill for the efficient practice of medicine, surgery and midwifery'. The Merrison Report recognized that this is no longer realistic.

This requirement has dominated the curriculum and examinations for medical degrees during the whole of my life as student, teacher, and examiner and merits closer scrutiny. For, although it is hoped it will soon be obsolete and succeeded by a new Medical Act, that time has not yet come.

The Act has never been a realistic one during my own experience which goes back over fifty years in clinical medicine. Its strict interpretation meant that on graduation the doctor was competent to perform any surgical or gynaecological operation, to deliver a child with the most difficult presentation, diagnose and treat the rarest poisoning, manage the most complicated medical, psychiatric, or paediatric problem. And examiners required such evidence as a written paper or a viva could provide that the student possessed such competence.

Two anecdotes may make clear the absurdity of the position.

A colleague, and a most distinguished thoracic surgeon, related how, during a locum in general practice soon after qualification, a patient told him she was being poisoned by her husband with arsenic. After consulting his books, he considered this to be possible. As a student he had performed Marsh's test for arsenic poisoning, and set out to repeat it on samples of her hair and nails which he duly collected. He found a flask, a funnel, some corks, and some glass tubing in the doctor's dispensary and made a suitable porcelain container out of a broken crucible. He got some zinc off the roof and set up the apparatus so that hydrogen could be passed over the heated nails and hair and so that the sublimed arsenic could be seen on the glass tube as he had been taught to do. He lit the hydrogen escaping from the tube at which the whole apparatus exploded. Fortunately he was uninjured. But he wisely asked the forensic laboratory to perform the next test.

During my tenure of the Regius Professorship at Oxford we reformed the teaching and examinations in some subjects. One was anatomy, at that time the student's greatest bug-bear in the development of his mind. We sought an examiner who would understand that anatomy was being taught as an educational subject and not simply for the practice of surgery. I thought I had found such a man in an old colleague. I listened while he asked the student to name the successive branches emerging from the abdominal aorta in a cadaver. When we got to the inferior mesenteric he asked what viscera were supplied by that vessel. The student gave a complete and correct answer but did not know the exact amount of the rectum supplied. The examiner asked me what I thought and I said that I thought he was very good, that the only question he had muffed was the last which, in my opinion, was trivial. No, said the anatomist, by no means trivial. You have to know that before you can excise the rectum safely. My mind still boggles at the thought of a newly graduated doctor undertaking the total excision of rectum on the faint remembrance of the anatomy he learned as a student.

These two examples show how absurd the literal interpretation of the Act now is. The fact is that the practice of medicine, surgery, and midwifery now requires such a range of practical experience that no man is ever competent over the whole. Perhaps the most important attribute of a competent doctor is that he knows what he can do and what he cannot do. The best doctors also know to whom to turn for help in a given case. The man who considers that he is competent over the whole field, whatever his previous experience and however many diplomas he has obtained, is a public menace. It is to be hoped that the new Medical Act will make postgraduate experience essential for practice and will not require competence in every subject.

I will say no more on this subject which is bound to receive the earnest attention of the General Medical Council.

2

The regulation of
medical education

Medical education in the United Kingdom is quite unusual in that
it is controlled not directly by Government but by a central
statutory body, the General Council for Medical Education (General Medical Council) established in 1858; and financed by the
Treasury through the University Grants Committee. Both the
GMC and the UGC inspect the medical schools through visitations, those of the UGC being at intervals of five years. The GMC
issues Recommendations (10) concerning the medical curriculum
(undergraduate) which medical schools should try to follow.
(Though, as we shall see, the 1967 Recommendations were too
'liberal' or 'enlightened' for the teachers.) The GMC may withdraw its recognition of a medical school as a 'licensing body' and
the UGC withhold funds if the teaching in a school is unsatisfactory. To date this has never happened.

In addition to the GMC's Recommendations, the pattern of
medical education has been greatly influenced by two government
sponsored reports, an Interdepartmental Committee of Medical
Schools (1944) chaired by Sir William Goodenough (4), and a
Royal Commission on Medical Education, chaired by Lord
Todd (5). The Government formally accepted the first and asked
the UGC to implement it. The Todd recommendations were not
formally accepted, but the University of London, the Ministry
of Health, and the UGC agreed to accept and to implement its
recommendations so far as they concerned London.

The Goodenough Report

The Goodenough Report was a most enlightened document. It
emphasized the importance of the university, of proper staffing,
of whole-time appointments, and of graduate education. It recom-

mended that there should be a compulsory year of house appointments before the licence to practise was granted, and that postgraduate training for specialists of four to five years should be organized. It recommended the abolition of the non-university schools in Edinburgh and Glasgow and their absorption by the university. The London medical schools were to become integral parts of the university and separate in organization and in finance from their parent hospitals. No new medical schools were to be established but if new ones were needed in the future they should be set up in existing universities. In view of overcrowding of hospitals in Central London, Charing Cross, St George's, and the Royal Free should move peripherally. Amalgamation of the smaller schools was not recommended.

Premedical training in medical schools should be abolished and transferred to proper university departments. Preclinical teaching should be shorn of unnecessary detail. In the clinical period, teaching should be organized by divisions of medicine, surgery, obstetrics, and pathology, each under the control of a whole-time university professor. Each division would have a full complement of whole-time university staff who in turn would have proper facilities for research and teaching. Honoraries who continued to teach medical students would receive a part-time salary provided that it was agreed that the professor was personally responsible for the organization of teaching in the division. The curriculum would be reorganized to make it a continuous whole, instead of a series of parts. Integration was the key word. To this end, preclinical and clinical studies should be pursued on the same site or as near to each other as was feasible and preferably on or adjacent to the university campus.

To put its proposals into effect it recommended that the Treasury should allocate an additional £1¾ million to £2½ million annually, and a capital grant of not less than £5 million. No school would be eligible for the new Treasury money unless it had agreed to effect the reforms in the report.

The implementation of the Goodenough Report was entrusted to the UGC on which I was privileged to serve at the relevant period (1944–54). I was fortunate enough to have two other experiences which increased my personal awareness of the change. I qualified at St Thomas's in 1928, joined the research and teaching staff of UCH in 1930, and became Professor of Medicine at St

Mary's in 1939. As Secretary of the Royal College of Physicians' Committee on Medical Education I wrote its report in 1944.

The Goodenough Committee considered that the optimum annual intake for a medical school was 100, for which a teaching hospital of about 1,000 beds was required. The Committee therefore encouraged the large schools of Edinburgh, Glasgow, Cambridge, and St Bartholomew's to reduce their intakes to this level, and the small schools in London and the provinces to increase. Teaching hospitals in general remained too small, but some universities like Edinburgh brought in the adjacent former municipal hospitals to help and planted in them whole-time staff of university clinical departments.

The Todd Report

The report of the Todd Committee published in 1968 may be considered under the following headings.

Postgraduate education. The Committee endorsed the changes that had occurred in the provision for an organization of postgraduate education since the fillip given to it in 1961 by the Nuffield Provincial Hospitals Trust (1), and the recognition of its profound importance. They thought no changes were required in the intern year, except that the universities should supervise it more strictly. This should be followed by a period of general professional training lasting about three years and embracing senior house officer and registrar posts.

> On completion of general professional training all doctors seeking a career in the hospital service should enter a single career grade of Junior Specialist. When they had the practical experience as a Junior Specialist they would be eligible for vocational registration and could expect promotion to specialist ... Promotion to the Consultant grade would be on demonstrated ability.

The period as a junior specialist would be occupied in advanced professional training of appropriate duration the details of which would be worked out, presumably by the universities, the Royal Colleges, and the NHS. Special arrangements would be made for training for general practice. In the assessment of general professional training 'there is no place for a single "pass or fail"

examination'. Assessment would be made on reports by supervisors.

> Some measure of objectivity will need to be introduced by
> using standard tests of knowledge and skill. If, as we hope,
> the early postgraduate period ceases to be dominated by
> preparation for formal examinations many more trainees
> should be able to take part in research ... The time has now
> come in our view for the establishment of a system of voca-
> tional registration as the necessary complement to a proper
> system of vocational training: we recommend that the Gen-
> eral Medical Council should be the vocational registration
> authority.

They considered

> there should be a central body to be known as the Central
> Council for Postgraduate Medical Education and Training
> in Great Britain for the general oversight of postgraduate
> education ... composed of representatives of the Universi-
> ties, of the main branches of the National Health Service
> and of the appropriate professional colleges.

Undergraduate education. They considered that 'the form of
apprenticeship in which the aspiring student walked the wards
with leading practitioners' represented 'an obsolete concept of
medical education'. The undergraduate course should be of five
years' duration, preferably offering a degree in medical science as
well as a medical degree, and including two years of fundamental
clinical education. The student should acquire 'first a knowledge
of the medical and behavioural sciences sufficient for him to understand the scientific basis of his profession', and secondly a
general introduction to clinical method and patient care in the
main branches of medicine and surgery together with an introduction to social and preventive medicine. They considered that
the undergraduate course should last five years, the preclinical
being increased beyond two years, and the clinical course 'should
be remodelled and reduced in length'. They favoured a three-year
preclinical course of a flexible nature based on modules. A possible curriculum, included two years of compulsory subjects, an
equivalent of one term on limited alternatives, and two terms in
two optional subjects. In addition to the present preclinical and

paraclinical subjects, the course would include epidemiology, statistics, evolution genetics, psychology, and sociology as compulsory subjects. The student would be able to qualify for a degree in medical sciences on completion of the course. In the clinical course they thought that the emphasis should be on collaborative interdisciplinary teaching such as the clinico-pathological conference, the clinico-pharmacological conference, the seminar, and the newer methods of integrated teaching and small group clinical teaching. They also thought that time should be found for the traditional clinical clerking and that this is of special value in an intensive, even if short, period of clerking during which the student is free of other commitments. Their specimen curriculum lasted 90 weeks.

> A course based on the principles outlined above would have no place for the kind of examination which has traditionally dominated the medical course ... The Medical Science degree examination would then consist mainly of a careful review of the student's achievement as shown by frequent reports or minor examinations in each module he has taken.

These assessments could be supplemented by an additional final test if this was needed to resolve any doubts about the appropriate class and degree. The same method would be applied to the degree in medicine built up from periodic reports on the student's performance based, where appropriate, on written oral or practical tests and completed by a comprehensive review at the end of the course.

The Report recommended an optimum size of 200–250 students a year as opposed to 100 by Goodenough. This important difference will be considered in the light of the experiences of the schools I have visited. They also recommended that the number of medical schools in London be reduced from twelve to six by a series of amalgamations and that each should become the medical faculty of a multifaculty institution. This again will be considered later in this Report.

General Medical Council

The Recommendations of the General Medical Council are, at least in theory, the basis on which medical schools plan their curricula for it is the Council that decides whether the degree of the university shall carry with it the licence to practise. The most recent recommendations of 1957 and 1967 both urged the medical schools to experiment. It is partly due to this that there is now so much difference between one school and another that it is difficult for students to change in the middle. Until 1970 it was quite easy for an Oxford preclinical student to proceed anywhere in the British Isles for his clinical work and for a clinical student from anywhere in the British Isles to complete his course at Oxford. The differences in curricula now make this virtually impossible. The last recommendations of the General Medical Council (1967) are so eminently in accord with enlightened university thought that I quote extracts.

1. The object of this basic medical education should therefore be to provide doctors with all that is appropriate to the understanding of medicine as an evolving science and art, and to provide a basis for future vocational training; it is not to train doctors to be biochemists, surgeons, general practitioners, or any other kind of specialist.

2. The Council feel that the primary task at the present time is to find means of reducing the congestion in the curriculum : to instruct less and to educate more.

3. The first fundamental requirement is that basic medical education should give the student knowledge of the sciences upon which medicine depends and an understanding of the scientific method.

4. The pursuance of study in greater depth in a selected area will not only bring the student into closer contact with the members of the staff but will allow him, with the incentive of his own interest, to learn to think scientifically in a field whose elements he has already assimilated.

5. The Council invites Licensing Bodies and Medical Schools to give consideration to the timing and form of their existing examinations, and to the possible use, to a greater extent than hitherto, of a system of progressive or continuous assessment throughout the student's career.

6. In reducing the load of the all-embracing final examination, it is important to avoid the hazard of burdening the

student with excessive and too frequent assessments. There may be a risk that in these matters of assessing and testing students a teacher will 'see and approve the better but follow the worse course'.

7. The Council considers that special weight should be given to the student's record throughout his course, and recommends that a system of continuous or progressive assessment should be established and maintained for this purpose.

8. The examination system designed by the University should aim at contributing to the education of the student. The primary object should be to test (and in doing so to foster) the student's understanding of what he has learnt and his capacity for thinking for himself, and not simply his factual knowledge.

Following a period of disenchantment with the General Medical Council, its functions, and mode of operation, a Committee of Enquiry into the Regulation of the Medical Profession was set up under Merrison (17). This Committee reported in April 1975. Its chief recommendations concerning medical education were that the General Medical Council should have control of all three phases: undergraduate training, graduate clinical training, and specialist training. It considered that a specialist education should be, in general, a precondition of the independent practice of medicine and that the control of the standards of specialist education should rest with the General Medical Council by its maintenance of a specialist register.

3

Postgraduate (graduate) and continuing education

The most important thing about education is appetite. Education does not begin with the University and it certainly ought not to end there.   W. S. *Churchill* (12)

The idea that education should continue after graduation is, oddly enough, a recent one in Europe. In the United States it took root much earlier, thanks to those great educators Eliot of Harvard and Gilman of Johns Hopkins, both, interestingly enough, scientists. In Britain, medicine is far ahead of other disciplines. Indeed, in Oxford and Cambridge the arts faculties are dominated by the concept that education ends with the first degree, and that, since the undergraduate course only lasts three years, the entrant must be well grounded in his special subjects, no matter the depths of his ignorance in the remainder (Pickering [13]). The idea of postgraduate medical education arose in many minds in the postwar period. The idea became a reality after the Christ Church Conference of 1961. As already noted, the impetus and the finance originally came from the Nuffield Provincial Hospitals Trust. Later the Ministry of Health (now the DHSS) provided most of the money, the universities the rest. Throughout, the Royal Colleges and Faculties have played a large part and, together with the universities, have set standards and enforced them.

A confusion of nomenclature should be noted. The term graduate student is often used for those studying for a higher degree (for example PhD) or diploma (for example FRCS) and postgraduate for later studies. But in medicine in the UK graduate student is seldom used. Postgraduate is used for all studies after the final qualifying examinations.

ORGANIZATION

Postgraduate and continuing education are organized on a regional basis, the regions being those corresponding to the old regional hospital boards and, since reorganization, to the regional health authority. Each region has a postgraduate committee whose executive officer, the postgraduate dean (or equivalent) is appointed and paid by the university. The committee consists of representatives of the university, the leading Royal Colleges and Faculties, the regional and area health authorities, the university appointed clinical tutors, and the regional adviser in general practice. Each specialty has a regional adviser appointed by the College or Faculty and usually a specialist sub-committee. One of the most important is that on general practice. The postgraduate deans and the clinical tutors have formed associations which meet several times a year as appropriate. Most of the finance comes from the DHSS through the regional health authority.

The work of the various regional postgraduate committees is co-ordinated by the Council for Postgraduate Medical Education in England and Wales whose report for 1971–5 (14) contains full details. The Council also advises about careers and runs career advice bureaux. The arrangements for Scotland are slightly different.

The postgraduate training of doctors is essentially an in-service training which may be considered under three heads: pre-registration house appointments; specialist training; and vocational training for general practice.

PRE-REGISTRATION HOUSE APPOINTMENTS

Compulsory pre-registration house appointments came into being in 1958 after the application of the Medical Act of 1953 (15). The approval of these posts and the assurance that the trainee is being properly educated during his period of service is the responsibility of the university, which is now usually delegated to the postgraduate dean and his committee. It is obvious that these training posts require a minimum of in-patients and out-patients, adequate supervision by a consultant and registrar or senior registrar, the provision of regular clinical meetings and post-mortem demonstrations and adequate library and lecture room facilities. Also there must be enough free time left over from service commitments.

The supervision of such posts by the university was initially so lax that a great deal of odium fell unjustly on the General Medical Council, and was partly responsible for the revolt against its authority. Since the institution of the postgraduate committees, the supervision has been well done.

The view is widely held, and I share it, that the pre-registration posts are not as good as they once were. This is partly due to the increase in number and the fact that a service now often has two house physicians or house surgeons when it used only to have one. Thus the responsibility for a complete knowledge of a patient is divided, with unfortunate effects on training. This adverse effect has been increased by the practice of the forty-hour week with extra duty payments for overtime—a concept that some of us older physicians and surgeons find incompatible with the ideal of service on which we embarked when we took up medicine as a career and entered a learned profession.

The increased output of medical schools since the growth of numbers fostered by Todd has led to considerable difficulties in providing enough house jobs. This is particularly true in certain regions. The solution will have to be a national one and is beyond the scope of this report.

REGISTRAR AND SENIOR REGISTRAR APPOINTMENTS

Training for specialties is largely 'in service', that is to say it is accomplished through holding posts in the NHS carrying a gradually increasing responsibility until, at the end, the doctor becomes a consultant and accepts full responsibility for his patients. This practice has developed gradually in British hospitals and was formalized by the Todd Committee into two periods, the period of general professional training and that of higher specialist training, each lasting approximately three years. The arrangements for such trainings are supervised by committees and have been set out by the Council for Postgraduate Medical Education in England and Wales.

The number and distribution of registrar and senior registrar appointments has developed piecemeal since the beginning of the NHS and now presents anomalies which will have to be put right. There is, for example, a tendency for consultants to regard senior registrars as their own private property. There is a conflict between the principle of a senior registrar being trained at a teaching hospital, because there he gets the greatest stimulus and the most expert supervision, and being trained at a peripheral hospital because there he gets the greatest volume and variety of experience. There is also a great disparity between the time which a doctor may expect to spend between beginning graduate training and reaching consultant status amongst the various specialties. These anomalies are recognized and steps are being taken to solve them. They are extremely important for the training of the specialist but are outside the scope of this report. The arrangements for in-service training vary much from region to region. In Birmingham, for example, trainee anaesthetists, surgeons, radiologists, and pathologists were assured, on appointment, of a succession of posts which would provide them with a full variety of experience. In other regions and in some specialties the trainee fends for himself with the advice of the regional adviser and postgraduate dean.

The supervision of specialist training largely devolved on the Royal Colleges and Faculties, though the universities collaborated. Where England and Scotland each have Colleges, as for example in medicine and surgery, joint committees have been formed to ensure uniform standards and practice. The supervision of specialist training involves the following procedures:

1. *The inspection and recognition of training posts.* This is done through the visit of an appropriate committee representing the appropriate College or Faculty, the postgraduate dean and representatives of the regional or area health authority. The committee looks particularly at the range and quality of work expected of the occupant, the degree of supervision, and the general facilities such as libraries and equipment. Since these committees usually include specialists who have come from a distance (to ensure impartiality) they have been difficult to arrange, expensive in manhours and in the money for travelling expenses. However, they have undoubtedly been of great value. In many instances the visiting committee would not recommend the recognition of the post for training purposes because of certain institutional defects. These had to be remedied if the post was to be recognized and thus attract a suitable field of good candidates. It is the intention that in future continued recognition of these posts shall be made through a less elaborate machinery, less expensive in consultants'

time. Probably the regional adviser in the specialty with the postgraduate committee will make the necessary recommendations, visitations being reserved for cases in doubt or dispute. Some regions, for example Wessex, have set up a Joint Advisory Committee for senior registrars. These visit strategic points in the region where they see each senior registrar on his own followed by the consultant on his own, and then the two together if necessary. In this way they identify problems on either side and hope to resolve them. In Wessex this is regarded as a very valuable and interesting exercise, but very time consuming.

2. *Enrolment of trainees.* In the case of most specialties, the trainee is required to enrol at the beginning of his training. His trainers are often required to report annually to the appropriate committee to ensure that the trainee's work is up to standard. If not, a visit from the regional adviser or some other member of the committee may be desirable.

3. *Assessment of fitness.* The criteria of fitness for specialty practice have been drawn up for the various specialties by committees representing the appropriate Colleges and Faculties, the Association of Clinical Professors (if any), and the various specialties. In general they specify the time spent in appropriate posts which shall have been recognized as suitable by the Faculties after visits by the appropriate accreditation committee. Reports of the graduate's performance in these posts may be required.

4. *Examinations.* All the Colleges and Faculties who participate in the training of specialists use examinations as part of the assessment of competence. These examinations in general test the candidate's knowledge of the underlying basic sciences, the phenomena of the diseases with which the specialty is concerned, and the detailed methods used in investigation and treatment. More and more, some knowledge of the epidemiology and social aspects of these diseases are required. Most of the examining Colleges have their examinations in two parts, the first including the so-called basic sciences and the second concentrating on clinical or practical aspects. These specialist examinations all have clinical examinations in which the candidate is presented with one or several patients on whom he is tested for his ability to take

a history, elicit the physical signs, and suggest further investigations and treatment, or he may have other appropriate practical tests as in anaesthetics, pathology, and surgery. He also has a viva. All use multiple choice questions to test the candidate's knowledge of fact or current dogma. Like so many other examining bodies the Colleges have become disenchanted with questions requiring long written answers. Indeed, the College of Physicians, that one time bastion of learning, now dispenses with any written evidence that the candidate can express himself lucidly and grammatically, can display evidence and argue from it, or is in the habit of reading, understanding, and critically assessing original papers. Exceptionally, the Faculty of Community Medicine demands a thesis and the Royal College of Obstetricians and Gynaecologists demands actual case records and commentaries of one obstetric and one gynaecological case containing adequate references to the literature.

As will be discussed in a later section, the questions asked in examinations are the only tangible evidence that the trainee has as to what his teachers consider important. Understandably, he believes that nowadays the leaders in his profession attach no importance to scholarly habits. This is the central tragedy of contemporary medical education. Such habits have made medicine into a highly respected learned profession and only the possession of such habits will keep it so.

5. *Certification.* Will be given by the appropriate bodies on completion of training. The recommended duration of specialist training (after full registration) are:

Anaesthetics: six years.
Community medicine: six years.
Medicine: not specified, but tending to be seven in all.
Pathology: minimum of six in all.
Psychiatry: seven in all.
Diagnostic radiology: five to six in all.
Radiotherapy: seven years.
Surgery: six to eight years, depending on the speciality.

FORMAL TEACHING DURING TRAINING
Most of the specialist Colleges or Faculties arrange appropriate courses particularly designed for its own diploma (membership

or fellowship of the College or Faculty). These courses are usually held at the College (particularly in Scotland) or medical school or at a postgraduate centre. Courses in the basic sciences are conducted in the universities and the Colleges. Where distances are too great such courses have been arranged at other centres, as in Wessex, before the University of Southampton Medical School was begun, and at Norwich. Frequently the trainee surgeon or obstetrician will hold a temporary post as a lecturer in anatomy which he may combine with a part-time junior clinical post. In this way, nearly every candidate who wishes it can acquire the knowledge of the basic sciences necessary for the specialist examinations.

Courses for the clinical aspects of the examinations are more widely available in appropriate medical centres. The responsibility for organizing these courses rests with the postgraduate dean and his regional committee advised by the specialist adviser in that subject who is an agent of the appropriate Royal College. Attendance at these courses by senior house officers, registrars, and senior registrars is facilitated by a day-release system. The expenses are covered by the DHSS. Teacher's expenses are similarly provided for, though the NHS consultant does not get a fee if the class is a ward round and part of his ordinary hospital duties.

The clinical meetings, clinical and pathological conferences, and grand rounds that are now such a prominent feature of all postgraduate institutes also help towards the education of the intending specialist.

CAREER GUIDANCE

An outstanding problem in specialist training is the disparity between supply and demand of the various specialties. For example, the NHS estimated that on 30 September 1971 the chance of a registrar with two or more years' experience getting a senior registrar post in the next year varied from 1 in 1 in mental handicap and child psychiatry and haematology to 1 in 29 in diseases of the chest. The chances were 1 in 6·1 in general medicine and 1 in 7·1 in general surgery. Certain specialties have become recognized as shortage specialties because of the difficulty in filling consultant posts. Amongst them are psychiatry, radiotherapy, pathology, anaesthetics, and diagnostic radiology.

In some of these specialties the difficulty arises because of the lack of suitable trainees, for example, geriatrics and psychiatry. In others the trainees are in great demand overseas, particularly in the United States.

My survey has shown that medical students are ill-informed about such matters. Both the English and the Scottish Councils for Postgraduate Education give advice on careers but the last pamphlet from the English Council was in July 1972 and the last figures were from the Ministry of Health on 30 September 1973 (in *Health Trends* [1974], vol. 6).

This important problem was discussed at Cambridge with the Postgraduate Committee and regional advisers. The suggestion arose that it would be useful to have an annual meeting of senior clinical students when the current state of career opportunities could be displayed. This would, of course, require an annual return of the relevant information by the DHSS. Neglect of this important matter may lead to an avoidable loss of medical graduates from this country.

General comments on graduate education

ADVANTAGES

The aim of the arrangements is to ensure that every graduate should be exposed to the right sequence of posts under the right conditions for training and that due credit should be given for having performed them satisfactorily. Also that an opportunity should be provided to attend formal courses given by competent teachers to provide the necessary theoretical knowledge on which specialist knowledge is based. These objectives have largely been achieved. In every region which I have visited, the dean, the postgraduate advisers, and the postgraduate committee were all agreed that their region provided opportunities for specialist education which should make an intelligent graduate into a competent specialist, provided that he had the initiative and enterprise to do the work, and that he knew how to learn.

DEFECTS

1. *Use of language.* Most overseas graduates and some of our own have a very limited appreciation of the use of language. They misuse words whose meaning they do not understand and they

cannot construct grammatical sentences. As a result, information is not accurately conveyed to them either in speech or writing; nor can they convey it to others. The seriousness of this defect is difficult to over-emphasize. An accurate history provides most of the information needed to manage any case in medicine and nearly all in psychiatry and is essential in every specialty dealing with patients. Failure to use language precisely means the passing on of misleading information from doctor to patient and from one doctor to another. This is the chief reason why the failure of examinations to test the use of language in both undergraduate and graduate periods is to be so deeply deplored.

2. *Concentration on examinations.* Many of the courses provided are unashamedly designed to ensure that the candidates can answer multiple choice questions and similar examination tests. Very few trainees are to be seen in the libraries and those mostly reading textbooks, such cram books as *Aids to Postgraduate Medicine* and *Aids to Undergraduate Medicine*, and the throw-aways which cater for examinations.

3. *Lack of time.* Most trainees and many teachers complain bitterly that the load of service requirements leaves little time for teaching or being taught. The head of a department of anaesthetics had to tell his surgical colleagues that on a certain day of the week there would be no, or a greatly reduced, service because the trainees would be engaged in a day-release training scheme. An out-patient clinic without teaching may deal with twice as many patients as one that does have teaching. Not many patients and too few administrators understand this conflict.

4. *Distance.* The time taken by both teachers and taught to travel to the centre where classes are being held may be a major obstacle. The steady growth of postgraduate centres has reduced this difficulty.

5. *The huge expense in terms of time and money involved in approving training posts.* The first report of the Joint Committee on Higher Medical Training recommended that every post should be scrutinized by a visit of three physicians, including one from a different discipline plus the postgraduate dean or his represen-

tative; a total of six doctors were initially required to approve every post for general professional training. Experience has shown that not all this number is required nor is the frequency of visits necessary. Too many distinguished doctors rightly resent the amount of their time and energy so consumed.

6. *Rigidity of training.* As in many aspects of life in the UK and particularly in medicine, an undesirable rigidity has crept in. The chief culprit is the necessity for the trainee specialist to register as a particular kind of animal at the beginning of training and to continue in that specialty. This is done to ensure a fully competent specialist at the end. But it has three major disadvantages:

(*a*) When a doctor's knowledge and interest is limited to a specialty he is liable to practise bad medicine. A patient who finds himself in his care with an erroneous diagnosis will have a very unfortunate experience, as I have witnessed in the past.

(*b*) There is no more certain method of arresting the progress of knowledge than to erect barriers and enforce them. Sherrington, James Mackenzie, I. P. Pavlov, and Thomas Lewis, to name a few examples, would not have made their unique contributions had they not strayed from one field to another.

(*c*) It is difficult or impossible for a university department to pursue a line of work if it does not fit a specialty. A professor of medicine who has illuminated the subject of fever, that common and obscure manifestation of disease, does not feel justified in asking any medical graduate to work in it because it conforms to no specialty training. This particular danger is formally recognized.

Thus the Joint Committee on Higher Medical Training (Second Report, 1975) states:

> It is not intended, nor is it possible, to lay down rigid prescriptions for the training of specialists. Any suggested framework in the following schedules should be interpreted flexibly.

The Joint Committee on Higher Surgical Training

> is unanimous in its desire to allow, indeed to encourage, initiative and independence.

Alas, the trainee judges his future prospects too important a matter to depend on the whim of a committee. Thus whatever the committee may do he is inclined to play safe and follow the strict letter of the law. Thus is his enterprise and originality suppressed. Moreover, those who interpret the rules are often less liberal than those who made them. Compulsory uniformity is a social disease from which medicine has not escaped.

The rigidity which has developed as a result of the recommendations of the committees on higher specialist training is having a disastrous effect on our ablest young graduates, particularly those in university service and who are interested in research. Not surprisingly, the more adventurous find in these recommendations one more reason why they should seek their intellectual and material fortunes outside this country.

It is very much to be hoped that this rigidity will now be ended. In my view, little or nothing would be lost by dispensing with enrolment in a particular discipline. Promotion and appointment to posts in the hospital service and university service in this country has hitherto been made without enrolment. I am not acquainted with any defects that have arisen and I can see nothing but harm arising from the proposed changes which seem an unnecessary example of bureaucratic interference.

Vocational training for general practice

About 40 per cent of doctors practising in the UK are engaged in general or family practice—primary care as they call it in North America. General practice is quite different from other specialties which are hospital-based, in the conditions of work, type of illness seen, and the advice and treatment most often needed. The general practitioner has a list of patients, usually families, whose medical needs he has to satisfy and who may call him at any time for consultation if they are, or think they are, seriously ill. He usually practises in partnership with one or more other doctors who not infrequently have special interests, the aim being for the partnership to embrace most of the common specialties. He may practise from a surgery in his house, but increasingly partnerships use health centres custom built for the practice. These health centres may contain, in addition to consulting rooms and waiting room, a room for records, and in the most up-to-date ones, a small laboratory, a treatment room, a small X-ray set, and an ECG and a dispensary. They may employ a social worker, secretaries, a record clerk, technician, and nurse.

Before the last war, general practice was the Cinderella of medicine. Many doctors used to take it up as soon as they were qualified and on the Medical Register, without doing any hospital jobs and thus having no postgraduate experience. Frequently, too, those who aspired to consultant jobs in medicine or surgery and who failed to secure advancement and who, in Lord Moran's unfortunate phrase, 'fell off the ladder', took up general practice. The rise in the competence and status of general practitioners is one of the encouraging stories in UK medicine. It owes much to the so-called General Practitioners' Charter of 1966 which brought better pay and secured financial allowances for ancillary help and made provision for help for health centres as the centres of general practice. Oddly enough the concept of the health centre goes back to the report of the Committee chaired by Lord Dawson (16) over fifty years ago and not implemented until recently.

Vocational training for general practice is a comparatively recent growth, and again owes much to the pioneering support of the Nuffield Provincial Hospitals Trust. It now receives much stimulus and guidance from the Royal College of General Practitioners, who have produced an excellent guide, *The Future General Practitioner, Learning and Training* (1972).

A number of schemes for vocational training have been tried out in England and Wales and Scotland. A more or less definite pattern is beginning to emerge. The course lasts three years. The first and last six months are spent with a trainer in his or her practice. During that time the trainee participates in the work of the practice, and meets regularly with his trainer to discuss interesting or difficult cases. The trainee will frequently ask his trainer to see a patient and vice versa. One day a week, or one half-day a week, the trainees in a particular town or district meet together, usually with a teacher, to discuss a topic chosen by them collectively. They are also encouraged to read in the library.

The remaining two years of training are spent in holding selected jobs in hospital, usually in the SHO or registrar grade. These were originally part-time and supernumary. But it is increasingly realized that trainees learn best by doing. What is learned when the trainee is to some extent responsible, is far more than what is learned when he has no responsibility.

The provision of jobs in the SHO and registrar grades for general practitioners was not easy at first. Hospital physicians and surgeons were used to training future specialists. But the support of the DHSS and the local postgraduate committees is gradually enabling the new system to prevail. The most popular specialties are ear, nose, and throat, psychiatry, general medicine, and obstetrics. Special arrangements are made jointly by the Royal College of Obstetricians and Gynaecologists and by the Royal College of General Practitioners for the training of those general practitioners who wish to practise obstetrics. There is an increasing number of GP maternity units in district general hospitals.

General practitioners are encouraged to take the examinations for the membership of the Royal College of General Practitioners. This diploma is not, however, necessary before a doctor establishes himself in general practice.

I have been greatly impressed with the enthusiasm of both teachers and taught in the schemes, with which I have become familiar in the course of this survey. They are producing a new breed of general practitioner which, in my opinion, will be much superior to any other anywhere in the world, and of course much better than their predecessors. I also had the opportunity to see something of schemes of training for primary care in the United States. These tend to be based on universities and teaching hospitals and not on family practice and are, in my opinion, inferior to those that have been developed in this country.

Postgraduate medical centres

These are mostly situated at district general hospitals where they serve as a focus for the intellectual and social life of the doctors and other NHS workers of the neighbourhood. From their beginnings in 1962 they have proliferated until in January 1977 they numbered about 300. They range in size and cost from the lavishly equipped and custom-built Cripps Centre at Northampton which cost £250,000 in 1972, to a couple of rooms set aside in a disused part of a hospital as at Amersham and Newmarket at the time of my visit; there wartime huts have been converted for the purpose. The most splendid of these centres have been provided by benefactions from philanthropic well-wishers. Many are the result of a drive for funds organized by the local doctors. Some have been provided mainly by the hospital authorities with small contributions from the university funds through the local Postgraduate Committee. Whatever its size, each of them has a library which may also serve as an office for the clinical tutor and the secretary and a lecture room which may also serve as a seminar room and common room. The larger centres have a dining room, a bar, a lecture room, a smaller room for seminars and tutorials, a library, an office for the clinical tutor and secretary, and suitable lavatories and cloakrooms. A car-park is essential.

In Scotland the movement towards postgraduate centres started later than in England. They are fewer, on the whole smaller, and many of them do not have a bar.

The typical postgraduate centres arrange to house:

1. Meetings of the local Medical Society, the local branch of the British Medical Association and the College of General Practitioners which usually provides lectures, demonstrations, and seminars for all kinds of doctors.

2. The classes arranged by the advisers in the specialties for junior medical or surgical training and higher medical and surgical training.

3. Classes for the primary FRCS and related examinations.

4. Clinico-pathological conferences.

5. Journal clubs.

6. Meetings of other societies, such as art and history societies.

The Dudley Road Hospital Postgraduate Centre in Birmingham has introduced an introductory course for new medical staff, giving them a tour of the whole hospital, explaining how the hospital is run, including the specialist servicing departments, for example, X-ray, pathology, etc., and the policy and mechanism for admissions and discharges and patients' records. This increased efficiency and the contentment of the staff.

An interesting example of local enterprise was seen in the Postgraduate Centre at Peterborough where a symposium on 'Stress in Industry' was organized by the clinical tutor at the suggestion of the Bishop's chaplain to industry. The participants included a psychiatrist, a personnel director, an industrial medical officer, and an industrial psychologist.

The frequency of the meetings and the numbers attending them vary very much from one centre to another according to local enthusiasm. This depends partly, but not entirely, on the enthusiasm of the clinical tutor and the secretary or librarian and the various organizers of the meetings and courses. The personality of the secretary or librarian (usually a lady) is a key factor in success or otherwise. In some centres meals are available through the hospital kitchen, in others local ladies (often doctors' wives) provide food and cook it. From time to time a pharmaceutical house will provide an exhibit and libations before and during the meal. The programme of an active centre is given in Appendix II.

To ensure good attendance, certain points have proved to be important.

1. That the visiting doctor should be made to feel welcome.

2. That the meetings should be arranged at times convenient to the majority of doctors concerned and they should be at the same time every week. The doctor can then arrange his work so that he can attend.

3. That, as well as having visiting speakers, it is very important that the doctors of the district should themselves contribute by presenting cases and by taking part in the discussions.

4. The provision of creature comfort, for example an appetizing meal and the products of a bar, make the occasion an enjoyable one, as well as intellectually rewarding.

The development of postgraduate centres was due to the initiative of the Nuffield Provincial Hospitals and is one of the success stories of British medical education. They have greatly raised morale in the hospitals and surrounding districts. It is therefore much easier to attract and to keep able staff. An example was given at the Dryburn Hospital, Durham, where they have a small but active Postgraduate Centre. Six miles away is Chester-le-Street which has none. The morale is much higher at Dryburn and the possibility of getting junior staff much better at Dryburn. This example could be repeated many times up and down the country.

There are, however, some outstanding issues. These are:

1. The attendance of consultants, junior hospital doctors, and general practitioners varies very much from one centre to another and from one individual to another. A good attendance of junior hospital doctors can be assured if the lecture or course is one that will help them with their next examination or one that the young person feels will advance him professionally. General practi-

tioners attend principally because they are interested and enjoy
it, and partly because attendance at five sessions per annum, approved for the purpose by the postgraduate dean, ensures seniority payments and postgraduate training allowance under Section
63 of the Health Services and Public Health Act of 1968. About
a third of general practitioners attend no more frequently, about
a third attend usually, and about a third are intermediate. Attendance is facilitated by the physical factors such as distance, times
of meetings, car-parking, and social amenities. In the last instance
it depends on the doctor's appetite for this kind of educational
experience. On the whole the younger doctors who have recently
emerged from an educational atmosphere attend more frequently
than older doctors who never had this experience since they finished their undergraduate medical course and then they did not
like it much. Although it is inherently probable that the excel-
lence of a doctor is related to the frequency of his attendance,
some of the best doctors have little time to spare from their
patients and prefer to study in the privacy of their home.

Apart from the provisions of Section 63, what has been said
for general practitioners applies to consultants. The two factors
favouring attendance are appetite and time. It is one of the sadder
aspects of recent developments in the NHS that the decline in
morale, consequent on the so-called reorganization with its multi-
plication of committees, and the unwisdom of the penultimate
Minister, has diminished enthusiasm and produced an enormous
waste of doctors' time. I never cease to find it astonishing that this
could have happened.

2. Financial rewards: the organization of courses and lectures
is time-consuming and is often unpaid. When the morale of the
NHS was far higher, this was relatively unimportant. Not so now.

3. Use of the library: in the Oxford region one of our small
district postgraduate centres carried out a survey of the use of
journals during one year. The most popular ones were the 'throw-
aways' like *Up Date, Hospital Medicine, Modern Medicine,* and
Medicine. These journals cater particularly for young doctors
preparing for examinations and are unashamedly vocational, but
the articles are well written and are equally favoured by busy
practitioners. The next most popular were the *British Medical
Journal, The Lancet,* and the *Postgraduate Medical Journal.* Virtually unread were some of the specialist journals, even I regret

to say, *The Quarterly Journal of Medicine*. I have enquired of librarians and inspected what people are reading on my visits up and down the country and the pattern revealed in this small survey seems typical of the country at large. This raises the question whether small centres should subscribe for specialist journals. Policy will have to steer a course between the advantage of continuity on the one hand and changing local demand as personalities change with retirement and recruitment. However, it does emphasize the importance of a regional inter-library service. Most regions provide this, so that at any centre a book or volume or a number of a journal can be got quickly and usually on demand.

The appetite for reading in the library and thus keeping up to date is seldom acquired after a man sets up in practice. It is most easily acquired in youth and again emphasizes the importance of undergraduate education.

Continuing education

This, too, is a comparatively novel concept. The French call it 'l'éducation permanente' which is better, for it describes precisely what is meant. It means, of course, that education continues until the grave or until senility makes a man unable to manage affairs. Whatever his specialty, it is of the greatest importance to humanity that a doctor should be up to date. It is, of course, impossible for him to know the latest developments in every subject for the advance of medical science is now progressing so fast that even if a man were to devote the whole of his time to it he would be defeated in his object. And, of course, the doctor is, or should be, busy attending to his patients. Nevertheless, whatever his specialty he should be aware of the general trend of developments so that even if they are outside his specialty he can insure that his patient is referred to someone who is more up to date than he is in that matter.

The means by which a doctor keeps up to date are three:

1. Reading current journals and books, which many doctors do in their homes, an opportunity which is widened by the libraries which are one of the conspicuous advantages of the postgraduate centres.

2. He may attend lectures and discussions which are provided by the postgraduate medical centres.

3. A most important part is the consultation through which he seeks the opinion of a colleague on his patient.

Self-respect is perhaps the most important component of happiness. The fact that all doctors are now able to keep themselves more or less up to date enables them to keep their self-respect and is thus a most important component of the morale of the NHS, which improved conspicuously until its peak in 1966. The decline in morale since then is due to unwise measures which lie outside the scope of this report.

Postgraduate medical education in Scotland

The NHS and its associated postgraduate medical education is organized differently in Scotland than it is in England and Wales. Scotland has about a tenth of the population of Great Britain and about a fifth of the medical school places. The teaching hospitals thus play a significantly greater part in the NHS in Scotland than in England and Wales. Moreover, the Royal Colleges in Edinburgh and Glasgow provide excellent teaching and library facilities. There is thus less need for postgraduate medical centres, except in Inverness which is the only one which is custom-built in Scotland.

There are five regional committees formed in 1970 in Aberdeen, Inverness, Dundee, Edinburgh, and Glasgow. Inverness has a director, the remainder postgraduate deans. The regional committees have representatives of the Colleges, the local university, the NHS, and the Scottish Home and Health Department. The work of the regional committees is co-ordinated by the Scottish Council for Postgraduate Medical Education whose composition is given in the footnote.[1]

1. The Scottish Council is basically tripartite in composition, that is, it directly represents the universities, the Royal Colleges and Faculties, and the NHS. It is composed of one representative from each University, one from each professional Royal College or Faculty, and one each from the University Grants Committee, the British Medical Association, the Scottish General Medical Services Committee, Hospital Medical Services Committee, and Hospital Junior Staffs Committee. The exceptions to the unitary rule are the Royal College of General Practitioners and the Secretary of State for Scotland, each nominating two members. The NHS is represented by six chief administrative medical officers drawn from the fifteen health authorities in Scotland.

Despite the paucity and late development of postgraduate centres, postgraduate tutors (the equivalent of clinical tutors in England and Wales) have been appointed by the universities for most hospital groups. These tutors work closely with the postgraduate dean in the provision and co-ordination of courses for postgraduate diplomas, for vocational training in general practice and other specialties, and for the continuing education of all doctors in their localities.

I was assured by the postgraduate deans in Edinburgh and Glasgow and by the secretary of the Scottish Council for Postgraduate Education that arrangements in Scotland are at least as good as in England and Wales and in general the medical graduate is provided with adequate facilities both in his training post and in his access to formal courses so that he can acquire the detailed knowledge and skills needed to practise his speciality.

4

Undergraduate education

The mind does not need filling up like a vessel but merely kindling like fuel.   *Plutarch* (17)

Is it not the great defect of our education today that, although we succeed in teaching our pupils subjects, we fail lamentably, on the whole, in teaching them how to think? They learn everything except the art of learning.
Dorothy L. Sayers (18)

In 1944, the year of the Goodenough Report, the undergraduate period was the whole of formal medical education; the graduate then picked up what he could by doing hospital jobs. In too many cases the doctor did no house jobs and steadily forgot his small store of knowledge which, because of inertia, lack of opportunities, and lack of incentives, he never refreshed. The attic full of unopened *British Medical Journals* was not unusual at that time.

The undergraduate curriculum attempted to cover the whole field of medicine, surgery, and midwifery, together with the basic medical sciences, pathology, public health, and forensic medicine; the student's knowledge was tested by a series of examinations in which the failure rate was of the order of 50 per cent. Cramming for examinations was the rule. Once the examination was over, the student emptied his mind of what he had learned, and prepared to take in a new supply, preferably in such a form that when he regurgitated it, his examiner would be satisfied. So-called factual knowledge was the order of the day, although as the Dean of Harvard, Sydney Burwell, told his pupils

In ten years' time, you will discover that half of what you were taught has proved to be wrong; and neither I nor any of your teachers know which half.

Writing in 1944, the Royal College of Physicians' Committee

on Medical Education (19), of which I was secretary, concluded that

> the average medical student has defects which are to be attributed chiefly to the manner of his training. He tends to lack curiosity and initiative; his powers of observation are relatively underdeveloped; his ability to arrange and interpret facts is poor; he lacks precision in the use of words. In short his training, however satisfactory it may have been in the technical sense, has been unsatisfactory as an education.

During the thirty years or so of professional life

> his ability to learn from his experience and that of others and to keep abreast of the stream of advancing medical knowledge depends entirely on those qualities in which his training has left him defective.

Today the situation is greatly changed. As we have seen, the opportunities offered to the young doctor in the graduate period are such that he can acquire all the specialized knowledge, techniques, and skills necessary for the practice of his specialty, provided he has learned how to learn. This then has now become the chief function of the undergraduate period and will become so even more when graduate education is legally required for independent practice. Therefore the outstanding issue for this part of my report is to discover how far the undergraduate period improves the mind of the student in curiosity, awareness, precision of thought and expression and in methods of collecting and assessing evidence which will enable him to reach a judgement. As we shall see many schools have hardly begun to achieve this object. Some few are well on the way.

Quality of students

Perhaps the outstanding feature of contemporary medical education in Britain is the high quality of students (14). In every university, medicine is by far the most sought-after faculty, and therefore receives the most gifted students. In the past the shortcomings of the average medical graduate could be attributed to low intellectual quality; today such faults as he has can be justly attributed mostly to his education.

Size of school

The Goodenough Committee recommended an entry of 100 students per annum as the optimal size for a medical school, with a 1,000-bed teaching hospital. Todd recommended 200 with a 2,000-bed hospital

> The school's complement of staff must be big enough to cover the main branches of the subject and to provide a strong intellectual community.

> We think that the provision of the complex and expensive facilities required in a medical school in future cannot be economically justified for those with an annual intake of less than 150 to 200 medical students.

> Wherever possible an annual intake of 150 to 200 should be aimed at.

> Schools which can take more should be encouraged to do so.

Between the two wars the University Grants Committee aimed at the Goodenough target. Since Todd, schools, except those in London, have been encouraged to expand. The largest is Manchester, with an intake of 200 into the preclinical school, plus, in the clinical years, a present intake of 50 from St Andrew's, rising to 70.

Opinion in the medical schools I visited was overwhelmingly in favour of the smaller intake. In Birmingham a preclinical professor remarked that when the intake had risen above 100 per annum the character of the student body had changed; previously cohesive, it had broken into smaller groups. All teachers agreed that as the school enlarged it became less and less possible for teachers, particularly senior teachers, to know their students. Discussing clinical teaching Manchester submitted to the visiting University Grants Committee

> The size of student groups (11 or 12) is a source of continual vexation.

> The ideal number is thought to be 6 to 9. Most of the patients are loath to be the subjects for teaching to one group of students in the forenoon and to a second group of Final Year students in the afternoon.

In small specialized units ... since all the students must be channelled through, the staff are faced with a repetitive programme ... and the experience gained by students is liable to be perfunctory.

In Glasgow, with an entry of 200, the clinical academic staff considered an ideal entry would be 100, which they achieve by having two clinical schools (the Royal and Western).

As we shall see, one of the main contemporary issues is, should medical schools concentrate on providing teaching or learning? Teaching can be provided for very large numbers; learning is an active process which is galvanized by dialogue between teacher and pupil. It is learning that is lost with larger numbers. More over, medicine is unlike any other university discipline in that it depends on personal relations between doctor and patient.

Todd's reasons for the large school do not withstand critical appraisal. At the time of my survey, one small school, St Mary's, had four Fellows of the Royal Society. Apart from Oxford, Cambridge, and University College, London, the other schools, including the biggest schools, had less and usually none. Only one good reason can be given today, namely to ensure enough doctors to man the NHS. To supply enough for its region was the thoroughly public-spirited reason for Manchester going up to 270. Manpower needs are so controversial that, not having studied them with care, I shall refrain from comment.

TEACHING HOSPITAL OR DISTRICT GENERAL HOSPITAL?
Increasing size has meant that the old clinical teaching hospital no longer suffices for clinical teaching. District general hospitals are more and more employed. Here the postgraduate medical centre has been an unexpected blessing, since its library, lecture room, and other facilities can be used for undergraduates too, though this was not the original intention. Indeed, the Cripps Centre at Northampton was deliberately planned with bedrooms for students which are much sought after.

A differentiation of function is beginning to emerge. There are certain parts of their course where students have to be concentrated near teachers, particularly the introductory clinical course and topic teaching. For these the teaching hospital is used. But in the larger cities accessory hospitals may be close enough to the centre for them to be used too. I was interested to find that students preferred to do their clerking and dressing at rather crummy old former workhouse infirmaries (now called Public Assistance Institutions) than the shining up-to-date teaching hospital. In London students preferred Lambeth to St Thomas's, the Central Middlesex to the Middlesex, and Paddington General to St Mary's. In Birmingham they preferred clerking at Dudley Road to the Queen Elizabeth, and at Manchester they liked the Royal Infirmary least. The reason is simple: St Thomas's, for example, has highly specialized units and departments doing advanced work in a limited field. It has many research assistants, senior registrars, registrars, senior house officers, and house officers. Last comes the student, and he has begun to feel almost an intruder. At Lambeth, on the other hand, the patients were a sample of the local sick, the nurses were delighted with new company to relieve their monotony, and the medical officers delighted to have additions to their overworked pairs of hands.

Glasgow has virtually two clinical schools centred on the Royal and Western Infirmaries. Manchester has two centred on the Royal Infirmary and the South Manchester Hospital (former PAI); the Hope is an embryo third. Increasing numbers of schools send their students to peripheral hospitals in their final year, usually in pairs to individual physicians and surgeons. Newcastle and Southampton use virtually the whole of the final year in this way. The reports from the physicians and surgeons are used in the final assessment. This is true continuous assessment and some district physicians and surgeons know their students better than some of the official teachers.

The use of district general hospitals for teaching at Southampton was part of the deliberate policy of building the new medical school into a teaching region. Here the great disadvantage of London is displayed. During the war, London was divided into a number of sectors, each based on a teaching hospital which supplied the district hospital with its own staff and students. It worked excellently. The Middlesex–Central Middlesex unit is a remainder. The reorganization of local government and of the NHS has, however, broken down the communications between the Middlesex and the Central. A plan to revive the wartime sectors in the interests of undergraduate and postgraduate education, put forward by the London deans, was, alas, rejected by the DHSS.

The curriculum

The object of the undergraduate course has been succinctly stated by the General Medical Council in its recommendations of 1967.

> In medical education, there should be a single objective for all doctors up to the time of full registration, whatever their subsequent career. The object of this basic medical education should be to provide a basis for future vocational training; it is not to train doctors to be biochemists, surgeons, general practitioners, or any other kind of specialist.

Before the change wrought by the Medical Act of 1956, which made a year's resident house appointments necessary before registration, the curricula of the British medical schools conformed to a general pattern. There was a year devoted to premedical subjects: chemistry, physics, and biology, five terms devoted to anatomy, physiology, and biochemistry, three years to clinical work, with pathology and pharmacology being fitted in somewhere along the way. The whole lasted five years in addition to the premedical year, which was generally done at school in England, but not in Scotland. There were major examinations in anatomy, physiology, and biochemistry (Second MB) and in the clinical subjects, obstetrics and gynaecology, medicine, and surgery (Final MB), with pharmacology and pathology being fitted in in a variety of ways. The form of the curriculum and of the examinations were dictated by the Medical Act and the need during this time to ensure that the medical graduate on qualification was fit to practise medicine, surgery, and midwifery. This, as we have seen, was quite an unreal objective. The compulsory year's appointment paved the way to graduate education which has become a reality and will soon be obligatory for all doctors intending to practise medicine.

The General Medical Council in its recommendations of 1957 and 1967 urged the universities to experiment. The present curricula are the result of such experiments. The trends have been in three directions. First, a curriculum planned by a committee of teachers of all grades of seniority, representing most subjects; second, integration; and third, continuous assessment.

PLANNING THE CURRICULUM

Most schools have set up committees to plan the curriculum and keep it under review to ensure that it is as good as it can be. Usually this committee also plans the examinations, for curricula and examinations are interdependent. Sometimes this committee contains students; sometimes there is a separate staff–student committee which reports the reactions of staff and students so that the curriculum committee is informed of current opinion. Some schools, such as Newcastle, one of the pioneers (1962) are now engaged in their third reform; some, like Birmingham, are in the second; and the newer schools are digesting their first experiment. Some few hardly seem to have made any significant departures from the old pattern.

The important point about curriculum committees is that they take the control of student time out of the hands of heads of departments, so that obstinate professors can no longer demand so many hours of teaching time (the 'droit de seigneur' principle).

OBJECTIVES

Medical education in the undergraduate period should have two principal aims. The first should be to give the student a general conspectus or overview of the whole field of knowledge. Such an overview is essential to any doctor and is of great value even to the specialist research worker for he thus knows when his scientific discoveries may have a useful practical application. The second aim is to train the student's mind so that its range of awareness is increased and his ability to ask questions and to answer them is enhanced. It is most important that in this period the young person should learn to express himself lucidly and concisely. If he has not learned to do this on graduation it is doubtful if he ever will.

In practice, the chief danger is and always has been that one subject hogs the first objective, thus leaving no time and no energy for the second. That subject used to be anatomy. At present in this country it seems to be biochemistry. A professor once asked his colleagues if any of them knew of a case whose proper treatment had depended on a detailed knowledge of the Krebs cycle. The response was silence. And yet no-one would deny that understanding the Krebs cycle is quite essential for the understanding of how the body works.

In order to give the curriculum a purpose or direction, many schools have outlined objectives. A widely accepted example is that of Newcastle.

General intention. He should have developed an attitude to medicine which is a blend of the scientific and humanitarian.

Scientific method. He should know that conclusions should be reached by logical deduction, and he should be able to assess evidence as to its reliability and its relevance.

Professional standards. He should be imbued with the high ethical standards required of a doctor. He should have learned how to deal with patients and their relatives, with sympathy and with understading.

Human biology. He should possess a knowledge of the structure, function, and development of the human body; of the factors which may disturb these, and of the disorders of structure which may result.

Clinical knowledge. He must learn how to elicit facts from a patient. He should have a good knowledge of those diseases which are an acute danger to life, and of the more common disabling diseases. He should recognize the limitations of his clinical knowledge and should be prepared, when necessary, to seek further help.

Environment and health. He should understand the effects of environment on health and should appreciate the responsibility of his profession for the prevention of disease.

Continuing education. He should appreciate that medicine is a continuing education and that he has an obligation to remain a student and to contribute if he can to the progress of medicine throughout the whole of his professional career.

INTEGRATION
The familiar departments of a medical school, such as anatomy, physiology, etc., were necessary for the acquisition of knowledge

because most people are competent to explore only a small fragment of the frontiers of science. Most people are also competent to teach to an advanced level in only a limited sphere. But for the ordinary student, intending to practise medicine, this fragmentation of knowledge is a fundamental disadvantage. Living people are not examples simply of physiology or pathology, or of psychiatry or of single organs. To understand them, and what has gone wrong, the student must be familiar with the structure of the whole body and how the body and mind work in unison and how this unison is disturbed in disease. He ought to know something, too, about the structure of society and the part this plays in illness and health. In the old curriculum the student had to perform the synthesis himself, in which he was not always successful. The trend now is for the teachers to do it for him, at least in part. This is the meaning and significance of integration.

The easiest form of integration is separately between the clinical subjects on the one hand and the preclinical subjects on the other. Preclinical subjects are commonly taught in a building separate from the hospital and not infrequently some distance away. Preclinical teachers tend to live a life centred on the laboratory. Clinical teachers tend to live a life centred on the patient. They often talk rather different languages so the synthesis is much more difficult. Nevertheless, while there is death there is hope. The recruitment of young medical graduates to the preclinical sciences has introduced a new spirit of co-operation, based on a common language and common objectives.

The major difficulty in effective integration, and the breaking down of intellectual barriers between subjects, lies in the minds of the teachers. Teachers are creatures of habit. They have always thought of and taught their subject in semi-isolation. To abandon this is like wearing a new pair of shoes. All the irregularities and angularities have to be compressed into an unfamiliar mould.

SYSTEMS COURSES AND TOPIC TEACHING

The easiest way to effect some sort of integration is to plan the courses of instruction in such a way that parts of the body are studied at the same time in the departments of anatomy, physiology, pharmacology, and pathology. This is about as far as some medical schools have been prepared to go. A further stage which is becoming increasingly popular is to plan the course as a whole on a systems basis. Integration may be achieved by representatives of two or more disciplines participating in one teaching session or, alternatively, by careful timetabling of individual components within the course. The second is much the less exacting. The course would begin with the basic anatomy, continue with the physiology, then deal with the pathology, then the clinical manifestations and finally the treatment. In many schools the course would end by selecting some common disorder, for example ischaemic heart disease, and attempt to integrate into the teaching anatomical, pharmacological, pathological, physiological, and clinical aspects together with the social implications. The ideal form of integration in which more than one teacher participates in a session and in which the students themselves contribute is very exacting in teachers' time. It had to be largely or partly given up in such schools as Birmingham because of the time consumed in transit in addition to the actual time of the session. The more teachers participate, the more exacting it becomes.

Integration has disadvantages as well as advantages. It makes exacting demands on the teachers who have to be prepared to abandon their habits of having regular teaching times each week, and accept whatever the Teaching Committee ask them to do. The curriculum becomes extremely elaborate and having been initiated it is difficult to change. Moreover, it is difficult for the student to absorb the philosophy of a single discipline such as physiology and to appreciate how the structure of knowledge has been built up.

Thus the history of medicine and of medical science tends to be one of the casualties of integration. This is unfortunate because it is true to say that a man cannot fully understand his subject without knowing something of its history. Here is another example of the prevailing decline in scholarship.

An example from Newcastle is an afternoon devoted to obstetrics. An anatomist and physiologist discuss first the anatomy and physiology of fertilization and implantation, the placenta and placental function (lecture and demonstration). This is followed by a lecture from a physiologist on sex hormone and gonadotrophic excretion in normal pregnancy and upon the basis of pregnancy tests. The final session of the afternoon consists of a panel discussion and demonstration organized by an anatomist, a physiologist, an obstetrician, and a physician, dealing with physiological and anatomical changes in normal pregnancy and the puerperium, and the effects of pregnancy upon the cardio-vascular system, blood, renal tract, and breasts.

Topic teaching is extremely exacting in teachers' time. To be successful the topic must be carefully thought out and correctly staged. Each teacher must know exactly what he has to do and how long he has to discharge his task. Otherwise the session degenerates into a series of disconnected mini-lectures, often repetitive, and long outlasting the receptiveness of the student's mind. In some schools, for example, Birmingham and Nottingham, the travelling time taken by teachers coming from other hospitals or their consulting rooms has meant reduction in numbers of sessions to, say, one weekly, or even their total abandonment.

When topic teaching is well prepared and rehearsed, students love it. Unlike the lectures, it cannot be got out of an ordinary textbook. And if it is designed so that the presentation is brief and cogent and if enough time is left for student participation, then it is very stimulating and discussion continues outside the lecture. Seminars in which the presentations are by students are very worth while, as long as they are well done and not too frequent.

Range of today's curricula

The old curriculum set out to cover the ground, to acquaint the student with the elements of the subjects legally required by the GMC. Present curricula also set out with the same objective, but to a varying degree they also try to train the student's mind. These are to some extent separate exercises. In the first, the student's role is largely passive; in the second, active.

The curricula and examinations are at present undergoing a detailed scrutiny commissioned by the GMC who kindly allowed me to inspect the draft report while I was preparing mine. Since theirs is more comprehensive and detailed than mine could ever be, I shall not attempt to duplicate it. I have the advantage of having interviewed students, graduates, and teachers and thus am able to report their reactions to the education to which they have been subjected.

Covering the ground

This remains the dominant objective in all schools. The task has been, and is continually being, made harder by the natural growth of knowledge and by pressure to include new subjects in the curriculum. This pressure has been successful to the extent that in 1944 when I prepared the Royal College of Physicians' report, the medical student was exposed to fourteen separate departments headed by a professor. Today the corresponding number is thirty for the average school. Each professor tends to be convinced of the unique importance of his subject; he therefore presses for curriculum time and examination time. This makes medicine unique amongst university faculties. In my more uninhibited moods I used to liken professors in the faculty of medicine to a set of birds of prey, each determined to have his pound of flesh from the medical student; an important function of the dean was to protect him. Two examples of this pressure were met during the survey. In one university a group of young teachers asked to see us; their request was to recommend that medical students should be compelled to learn electronics, because of its increasing importance in medical technology. In another university the professor of geriatrics and the professor of general practice, both newly appointed, told us with delight how each had secured so many hours of teaching time in the curriculum. These then are the new pressures on the student. On the other side are the forces supposed to be working for his relief—integration and continuous assessment.

We may now enquire to what extent these have been put into practice and been successful.

Present curricula. My survey has revealed a great diversity. In those schools where clinical and preclinical schools are separated, for example, Cambridge, Cardiff, Glasgow, Oxford, and St Andrew's, the preclinical curriculum and the examinations are still organized on a departmental basis. In some, with integrated curricula, one or more departments remain aloof, for example, anatomy (St Mary's), biochemistry (Southampton), and pathology (Newcastle). Some, for example, Oxford, have not yet included social and behavioural sciences in the preclinical curriculum, believing they are adequately covered in the clinical period.

In a few schools, notably Newcastle (the pioneer), Nottingham, and Southampton, students are introduced to patients from the very beginning of the course. Students like this. Sometimes clinical demonstrations are used to illustrate anatomy and physiology. These can be most stimulating. Sometimes when teaching is based on systems, classes on form and function are followed by pathology and clinical aspects of disease of that system. This bringing together of different disciplines is also greatly appreciated by students.

The bridging of the gap between preclinical and clinical studies has been most successfully achieved by early introduction of patients to students and by including preclinical teachers in topic teaching in the clinical years. A relatively unsuccessful experiment was the so-called 'Bridge Course' at Oxford. The student fresh from his Final Honours School in physiological sciences came to the Radcliffe Infirmary and was at once given a four-month course based on morbid anatomy and its clinical implications, together with elaborately constructed topic teaching and an elementary course in history-taking and physical examination. It was subsequently agreed that this was an excellent course well constructed and well conducted but at the wrong time. The student who had been confined to the preclinical lecture room and laboratories for three or four years could not wait to deal with patients and felt utterly frustrated if instead of doing so, he was again asked to sit and listen to lectures. The course would have been admirable a year later in his curriculum. All schools have an introductory course in history taking and physical signs. The classes must be small and this is always a major problem in the larger schools. The mastery of such clinical methods is perhaps the most important objective of the clinical curriculum. Today it is mostly badly done. This requires more attention by teachers.

The clinical period reveals a similar diversity. From it I select two issues that seem to me the most important, namely, should teaching be confined or nearly confined to the teaching hospital, and should clinical teaching be mostly through apprenticeship or through lectures and demonstrations? The first has been dealt with. The second now needs attention.

The role of apprenticeship

Medical education in England has always been based on apprenticeship. After an introductory course, in which the student was taught how to take a history from a patient and to examine him clinically, he was appointed to a physician (clerk) or to a surgeon (dresser). He worked up the patients allotted to him under the supervision of the registrar and house physician, and was in a position to present the salient features of each patient to his chief when he visited the ward. This apprenticeship was supplemented by lectures and demonstrations.

At its best, clerking was an excellent education. The student's notes were read and commended or corrected. He discussed patients on equal terms with his teachers. He prepared his 'essay', read it to his 'tutor' and received helpful criticism: at its best, a good tutorial. He early experienced a very curious phenomenon of great importance in medical education—the so-called 'drop of the penny'.[1]

At first the medical student entering the wards is bewildered by the endless variety and complexity of the range of phenomena presented to him. In many people the replacement of chaos by order happens quite suddenly. In my own case I remember it vividly, just as vividly as Darwin remembered the moments of sudden illumination that characterized the development of his theory of evolution by natural selection. After this experience the medical student learns readily from each new patient he sees. If he has acquired clinical method in this way, his future as a clinician is assured.

Unfortunately clerking was not always like this. Too often the student's notes were unread and uncorrected. He seldom presented his cases to his chief who scarcely seemed to know him. Even the registrar and the house physicians were too busy to take an interest in the student. The teaching rounds became a collection of long white coats (doctors) whispering together round the patient, while the short white coats (students) decorated the periphery.

The alternative lecture demonstrations in which a junior or senior teacher selected a patient to demonstrate to, say, ten to

1. Named by Dr Donald Hunter of the London Hospital with whom I used to examine at Cambridge. Machines in piers and fun fairs required the insertion of a penny to make them work. When the penny dropped, the machines started up.

twenty students, was the preferred method of teaching in the Scottish schools, where student numbers were larger and where the influence of the European universities was greater: for in the great European universities clinical teaching was almost entirely by lectures and demonstrations, the classes being often over 100.

In the new curricula, the accent on integration and frequent examinations has emphasized teaching as opposed to learning and has diminished the importance of clerking. Nevertheless even in the most advanced examples like Newcastle and Southampton, clinical clerking plays an important part in the scheme of medical education. The success or otherwise of clerking depends absolutely on the physician or surgeon to whom the student is apprenticed, for the student tends to model his behaviour on that of a chief whom he respects. If the chief is interested in his student's work, encouraging him, applauding good work and deploring bad, then the student develops good clinical habits which will last a lifetime. The only other period of comparable importance in habit forming is that of the house appointment.

The consultant staff at teaching hospitals are supposed to be chosen, at least in part, for their academic standing, including their capacity as teachers. At district general hospitals consultants are not chosen on this basis. That does not necessarily disqualify them as teachers. Most of the London schools and many of the provincial ones send their students out to act as senior medical and surgical clerks (or unqualified house officers). They are able to select those posts where the chief is prepared to take trouble with his students to the profit of both.

Continuous assessment

The idea that a student's merit can be judged on his class work as well as by examination is familiar in the ancient universities. In Oxford colleges, each student is presented by his tutor to the Head of the college at the end of every term, and the reports of his supervisors read out. Some of these reports are virtually useless (for example 'satisfactory'), some are acute analyses of the student's work, of his merits and his failings and how his competence may be improved. That masterly document the Haldane Report on the University of London (20), said

It appears to us only fair that due weight should be given to the whole record of the student's work in the University.

To do this in medicine implies that at each stage in his education the quality and quantity of the student's work should be assessed. In the laboratory sciences this can be done in the practical classes and it can be done in seminars and tutorials. In the major clinical subjects like medicine, surgery, and midwifery it can be done when clerking and dressing is the basis of education. For example, I required my clerks to present their cases to me and this was the preferred method by which I took care of the sick. At the end of their three months' appointment I was pretty clear as to who were the excellent, the good, and the indifferent, and who had utterly failed to become interested or competent. This information could be added to and checked by the opinions of house physicians, registrars, and ward sisters. While this can be done in the major subjects in which each student is exposed to teachers for considerable periods, it is more difficult in minor subjects and in these assessment demands some sort of test.

It would clearly be ideal if examination could be dispensed with altogether (as in Yale Medical School)[1] and the adequacy of a student be judged entirely on his class work. In medicine in this country this has not yet proved possible because:

1. An accurate assessment of the merit of a student's work requires a great deal of time and effort on the part of the teacher. At Oxford I tried to get such a system initiated but my colleagues felt that the reports, particularly from some London schools on clinical students would be virtually useless because the teachers did not know their students. I maintained that that should be one of the objects of the reports—teachers should know their students' work well enough to write a report.

2. It is difficult to exclude personal bias.

3. Under the present Medical Acts the GMC would not feel able to dispense with examinations as part of the procedure conferring a licence to practise.

For these reasons continuous assessment has become frequent examinations. In one school there are now sixty during the five-year period. In most schools there are at least termly examina-

1. The Yale degree does not license to practise. In the USA there are separate examinations for the State Boards which confer this privilege.

tions and in many cases they recur at much more frequent intervals. As will be explained in a later section, examinations now tend to take the form of multiple choice questions in which the candidate is presented with a question, and a range of possible answers of which he has to choose one. Often the question papers require that he should identify the answers in appropriate spaces so that the answers can be marked mechanically. Many schools have adopted the laudable objective of replacing major examinations like the traditional Second MB and Finals with these 'mini' examinations. The argument advanced in their favour is that they encourage the student to work. But at what? Swotting up his textbooks and lecture notes so that he can regurgitate the answers to the questions he thinks he will be set? Many students consider, and I agree, that they have now become a tyranny. The student never has a long enough period free from examinations to develop and pursue an interest. However, the most serious effect of the tyranny is that it discourages scholarship. The hallmark of a university education used to be that the student was disciplined in the habits of scholarship. He was taught to consult the sources of knowledge, to quote the sources precisely, and to be able to display and assess evidence. On that evidence he would acquire the habit of basing a judgement or giving an answer. In modern medicine he is required to give the answer without the evidence, the very negation of scholarship. He is not encouraged to write and speak lucidly and grammatically. In fact he is denied the most important tools of learning.

The growing illiteracy of students is not therefore surprising. At one Curriculum and Examinations Committee when a student's failure to write good English was pointed out, a student remarked: 'It is not surprising since all we have had to do since we came to the university is put ticks in the right boxes.'

To assess worth on actual performance is, of course, difficult and much less numerically replicable than is the mechanical marking of a multiple choice questionnaire. To do it well requires much the same qualities as are needed in a good physician, namely the ability to listen with critical appreciation, and insight into character. Some people have these qualities and do it well. Others have not and do it badly. Because assessment of performance is so subjective, it is unlikely to substitute entirely for examinations; neither staff nor students would accept that. But assessment of performance can supplement examinations. For example, in Birmingham when I was external examiner, a student who had done badly in his examination was not judged a failure until his record had been produced and scrutinized. If his record was excellent he passed, unless his examination had been abysmal.

Judgement of worth by performance can have these merits which MCQs lack.

1. It encourages the student to work in a scholarly way and to master his subject.

2. It can and should test the student's knowledge and his ability to use it constructively.

3. It can and should test the student's ability to collect and display evidence.

4. It can and should test the student's ability to express himself both in speech and in writing.

Assessment of worth by performance is educational for both student and teacher. It cannot be done unless the teacher has been keenly interested in what the student has actually done. Like every other technique, assessment by performance can be improved by practice and by discussion, particularly between teachers and students. If it is done really well, it is the best test of a student's competence. Even if it is done less well, it encourages the teacher to take a real interest in his pupils.

Reactions to the present curriculum

For the vast majority of medical students in Great Britain the medical curriculum is virtually as it was thirty years ago—five years of similar teaching, modified by varying degrees of integration and punctuated by repeated small examinations and swollen by the addition of behavioural and social sciences. Both students and staff have very serious criticisms of this course, particularly in the first two years. The students in all the schools we visited, except for three, described the course as boring and themselves as frustrated.

We are treated as data-banks; we are expected to sit in a lecture theatre and write down what is said and then learn our lecture notes so that we can reproduce them for the next test. All we think of is the next test.

It is evident that in most schools the student is over-taught and over-examined.

Two comparisons were possible between the reformed and the unreformed curriculum. We met several Birmingham graduates, both at Birmingham and elsewhere, who said they were glad they had graduated before the new curriculum was instituted. They gave as their reason that the old curriculum left you free to develop and follow an interest. The new curriculum did not. At the Middlesex Hospital Medical School, where the new curriculum had been introduced shortly before our visit, a similar preference for the old was expressed, the reason being that the introduction of social and behavioural sciences had increased the demands made on the student in terms of teaching time and examinations, so that he was under constant pressure.

Two other student reactions may be quoted. The Birmingham students prepared a detailed critique of their course and examinations for us. This they eventually elaborated into a paper in the *British Medical Journal* (21). In this paper they made the following recommendations for modifying the course:

1. A core of essential knowledge should be defined and outlined clearly to students and staff, then used as the basis for examination and for defining the pass/fail border.

2. There should be more essay projects and tutorial work and fewer formal written examinations.

3. Various types of questions should be incorporated into each examination and less reliance placed on multiple choice questions.

4. Greater and faster feedback from staff is needed; there should be sessions to go through written papers and more discussion with essay supervisors.

5. The criteria used in clinical assessment should be defined more clearly.

6. Housemen and ward sisters should take part in assessments on the ward.

The Association for the Study of Medical Education held a conference at the Royal College of Physicians in London in December 1975. Mr Watt, a student from Aberdeen made these points.

> The curriculum that the speakers have been talking about has been very much a teachers' curriculum.

> When a student has qualified, it matters little what he has been taught, only what he has learned.

> That is very characteristic of British medical education, students being made passive recipients in an education process of spoon feeding.

Students had identified six problems in medical education: inability of teachers to teach and their ignorance of educational methods; student apathy in the face of poor curricula, repetition, omission, and irrelevance in the course; the lack of effective staff–student co-operation at all levels; autonomy and lack of co-operation between departments and the scarcity of educationists in the medical field.

Some of the more important criticisms of teachers are exemplified by those of the Executive Dean at Birmingham.

> The preclinical course is so elaborate that no part can be altered without the whole edifice crumbling.

> The curriculum is very demanding on the students, with far too little time left for self-education and thought. Not more than half the students' time should be consumed in set classes. The other half should be available for self-education such as projects, essays and reading in the library.

During my visit to Birmingham I toured the library between 4.30 and 5 pm. Seven students only were reading original papers. Three were doing a BSc (non-medical) course. One was a fifth-year student preparing the subject of cardiomyopathy for his chief (who was also reading in the library) and there were three medical students preparing their essay in pathology. Five medical students out of 600 (about 1 per cent) is a proportion similar to that I observed in other schools in the survey, except Oxford, where the essays set by the college tutors make the proportion much higher.

These criticisms of the undergraduate curriculum are very serious. I have carefully examined the evidence from timetables and from the examination papers and I have no doubt that they are substantially justified. Interestingly enough they are the same criticisms as were made (and justified) thirty-three years ago when the Royal College of Physicians' report was published. The causes and the remedies are the same and they have been correctly diagnosed by the students.

The chief cause is the attitude of the teacher. He is convinced of the importance of his own subject. He tends to see his subject in isolation, apart from all others. He is deeply convinced of his right, nay his duty, to ensure that the student can reproduce enough knowledge of it in examinations. This attitude comes most easily to those preclinical teachers without medical degrees, because to them their subject really does exist in isolation. This attitude, of course, is excellent for the progress of knowledge; it is the stuff of which the world of learning and of the universities has been made. And if there were only three or at most six subjects in the curriculum, as there are in every faculty except medicine, it would do no harm. But in medicine it is the student who suffers and who has been forgotten. Again, the teacher is convinced of the over-riding importance of factual knowledge. His teaching therefore tends to be a catalogue. The growth of MCQs emphasizes the importance of dogmatic statements, whether they are of established fact or the opinions of the relevant teachers and examiners (in the modern medical school with frequent internal examinations the examiners are necessarily identical with the teachers). Moreover, the display of evidence, *a fortiori* its collection, takes time, and there is no time. Finally, there is the vital problem of examinations. Informed opinion is agreed that MCQs are replicable. There are grave doubts as to whether tests of a candidate's ability to display evidence, and to argue from it, and to write lucidly and grammatically can be tested with similar precision. Therefore these qualities are not tested and the student is led to believe they are unimportant. This vital problem of examinations will be taken up later.

But surely, the reader will ask, have not the planning of examinations and curricula by committees remedied all this? It is plain they have not. Junior teachers are no wiser and no more familiar with educational methods than their seniors. Moreover, all teachers are creatures of habit; they tend to do to others what was done to them. 'Plus ça change, plus c'est la même chôse.'

The remedies

EDUCATION IN DEPTH

The remedies to end this sad state of affairs follow from the diagnosis as the students suggested. The remedies have already been applied in a few schools. They are: ruthless pruning of time-tables and a degree of education in depth with the substitution of active for passive learning. For the remaining reform, that of the examinations, the time is, alas, unripe.

In the last revision of their curriculum, the Southampton Medical School reduced teaching time from 22 hours to 20 hours a week. This would seem to be right. But it is difficult to achieve. A young man in his penultimate year at Cambridge has 34 hours of lectures and laboratories weekly, an affliction faintly mitigated by the term lasting no more than eight weeks. Pruning the time-table is one of the most arduous exercises in which a school can engage. The prize has to be substantial. It is. It is no less than the mind of the student as a thinking instrument.

The importance of education in depth as a medium for de-veloping the student's mind as an instrument of enquiry and pre-cision should need no emphasis. But unfortunately it appears that it does, so isolated from the general world of education has medi-cine become. Education in depth ensures that at least on one occasion in his life the student has become familiar with how knowledge has been built up, how the evidence has been won, how hypotheses have been born and have died as new facts have come to light. He learns the value of evidence from some of the celebrated scientific controversies in his chosen subject. Such an experience enables the student to set for himself a standard and to acquire a habit of mind which is essential for the development of his full mental stature. There was a time when the quality of students was so poor that to attempt to do this was a waste of time. Not so now.

For many years it has been possible in every university for a few medical students to take an extra year for an intercalated BSc, two years for an Honours BSc in Glasgow. Some of the best students have done this and have provided more than their fair share of the leaders of the profession. In Cambridge every student had to take an honours degree. But this was given on Part I of the Natural Sciences, or latterly, the Medical Sciences Tripos, which

was more like a glorified Second MB. Part II of the Tripos at Cambridge, and the Final Honours School at Oxford required a year
for a single subject. Thus at Oxford and Cambridge, as in other
universities, the year of study in depth is an additional year.
Nottingham has followed Oxford's example.

The idea that all students during their ordinary medical course
should have an opportunity of undertaking an original enquiry,
however small, and of writing it up in an acceptable literary
form suitable for publication, has been favoured by Newcastle
and developed to various degrees by Birmingham and St Mary's
among other schools. Some of these projects have resulted in
publications. But the idea has been developed furthest by the
new medical school at Southampton (Appendix III). Here the
fourth year is largely devoted to a project which the student se-
lects together with a supervisor. He devotes the whole of his time
to this for the best part of a year; but on one day a week he is
assigned to clinical duties. This new medical school has been going only long enough to graduate its first class, but my enquiries
have led me to believe that the GMC visitors and the internal
examiners are satisfied with their performance. How they will
perform in later life and how they will compare with other
graduates remains to be seen.

Nevertheless, I would like to hazard the opinion that this venture of Southampton's is the most important experiment in medical education in my life-time. It should provide the young graduate with the discipline and habits of mind of the scholar, and
thus fit him for the opportunities of self-education which he will
enjoy after graduating and for the rest of his life. And it can be
done without adding to the length of the curriculum. There is
only one doubt: can such a programme continue to be worthwhile or possible when numbers of students increase greatly?

ACTIVE AND PASSIVE LEARNING

I would agree entirely with the students that a major defect in
contemporary medical education is that too much passive learning is imposed and too little active learning encouraged. It is true
that the student who wants to can undertake a piece of original
work in his elective period. But the venturesome student will prefer the Grenfell Mission in Labrador, the Mission Hospital in
Zululand, or something in another exotic land, and the timid will

retake a course he thinks he has done badly. The great virtue of the project is that it requires effort on the part of the student. There is nothing that raises student morale as much as rewarded effort. This was illustrated at the ASME Conference in 1975 already referred to. Professor R. Crooks stated how, when he was at Aberdeen, he and his surgical colleagues wanted to know how many patients who had had gastric surgery developed bone disease. They assembled the fourth year, explained the problem, gave them a list of patients and £100 given by a drug firm.

> I have never seen a fourth medical year work so well and be so enthusiastic. The first thing they did was form a committee. They then had a dinner when they discussed their plans. They hired cars. They went out to the homes of these patients and brought them back in. They obtained blood samples and they interviewed and examined them. They detected the predicted 7–10% patients with bone disease. But furthermore they had started reading books. They found of course that iron deficient anaemia is a complication of gastric surgery, so without any supervision or direction they picked up 30% of patients who had haemoglobins of less than 70%. They then admitted some of the patients to hospital. They then wrote the paper and finding that they had about £30 left they had another dinner.

What a contrast to the boredom that was so commonly reported by the students and that was the most distressing finding of this survey.

The attitude of mind of the teachers

My survey has convinced me of what my experience as a Professor of Medicine had suggested, namely that far more important than details of the curriculum is the attitude of mind of the teacher. Learning is easy if it is a pleasurable experience and if the student finds the process interesting and exhilarating. The secret is simple. As I used to say to my young men, the function of the teacher is to get the student to do the work. His attitude should be that of kindling the flame rather than filling the pot.

The late Sir James Spence (22) once remarked that there were four instruments of clinical teaching.

1. *The lecture* which is a process of conveying information and ideas from the teacher to the taught. As long as the student can hear the voice and see the exhibits accompanying it, it does not matter how big the audience is. Television and the Open University make use of this. But the lecture must be well prepared and the teacher should descend to the level of his audience so that they can understand. I recently attended two advanced lectures in medicine. In one the lecturer recognized that many of his audience were not specialists like himself, and explained. The audience was entranced. In the other there was no such recognition and to most of the audience the lecture was incomprehensible. They were bored. Students react similarly.

2. *The seminar* in which a small group, up to twenty, sits around a table. They discuss a subject prepared by one of their number. This can and should be a student, undergraduate, or postgraduate. One of those taking part should be an expert, but there can be more than one, as in topic teaching at its best.

3. *The ward-round* where the teacher and the class concentrate on the presentation and discussion of a single patient or more than one. The problems of diagnosis and treatment are displayed and the group will discuss the relationship of the patient's occupation and way of life to the pathogenesis of the disease, and the influence of his home circumstances and his work on the management of the disease and, finally, the availability of social services to help.

4. *The out-patients' clinic* serves two purposes. It displays disease before it has reached the stage of hospital admission, or which will never reach that stage, and how to manage patients out of hospital. But it should also display the technique of consultation; for the patient has been referred by a general practitioner to whom the patient will be returned, with suggestions for further work in diagnosis, and how to manage the patient in relation to his circumstances.

The good teacher will understand the function of these instruments of teaching and use them in that way. But the best have something more. They require the active participation of the student. In ordinary clinical teaching this may be done in two ways.

The presentation of the patient. In my experience the most important achievement of the good student is the ability to work up an individual patient and to present his case lucidly and concisely to an audience, and discuss its importance, with a good appreciation of what is already known and what is unknown about the disease. That this method is disappearing from the average medical school is one of the saddest of my experiences. In far too many schools the students told me that they had never done this. The blame is to be laid on the individual teachers but also on the management of the school for not insisting that it is done.

Asking individual students to prepare a controversial subject. When, as frequently happens, the teacher and his audience cannot answer a question with assurance, a student can be asked to go and look it up and report back at the next session. It was his capacity to do this with his graduate assistants that made a former Professor of Surgery at St Bartholomew's so productive of good young men. In my survey I found one such student working to this end in the library, and only one.

Training the teacher

The medical students stressed the importance of training teachers to teach. I agree with them and would like to make the following points.

Various attempts have been made to improve the performance of teachers by getting professional educationalists to address them. Mostly these have been sterile. Professional educationalists tend to dwell on educational theory, and neglect what it is that makes a good teacher. Discussions have been organized at which distinguished medical teachers have talked to the young about the key to success as a teacher. These have not always been successful. I have attended two of these meetings in which the leaders displayed elementary mistakes, such as lecturing to the blackboard and projecting slides with either blank sheets of paper, or else so much data as to be unreadable from the back.

Most medical teachers model themselves consciously or unconsciously on their own teachers whom they have most greatly respected. Thus the Edinburgh school has been noted for having lecturers of great distinction and popularity and tends to produce such. I believe that each medical school should arrange for its staff and senior students to discuss the objectives of medical teaching and how they can be achieved. The vehicles of medical education and the way in which they may be used have been mentioned already. I would like to add these points. The best teachers are enthusiasts. Their enthusiasm infects their students. This is most likely to happen if the teaching is active and the student is urged to find things out for himself. The greatest crime of the educator is to bore the pupil. Sometimes a teacher is very successful in one medium and quite unsuccessful in another. A great lecturer may be quite useless in encouraging students to work on their own and vice versa. The wise dean will use his staff in the medium in which they are most successful.

Behavioural studies, community medicine, and general practice

Most schools have introduced teaching of these subjects into the curriculum with varying degrees of success.

At one extreme lecturers in academic departments of psychology or sociology have lectured to medical students. These in general have been a failure with the class being bored. There are two reasons. First, the lecturer's use of his own brand of jargon which the average medical student does not understand. Second, the student is anxious to see patients and feels frustrated by simply sitting in lecture theatres. At the other extreme the teaching is in charge of medically qualified personnel. They succeed in interesting the student, particularly when they arrange that he should go into the community; for example visits to prisons, juvenile courts, child guidance clinics, old people's homes, and factories. These visits are time-consuming to arrange and conduct but they pay handsome dividends in terms of arousing the interest of the student and in providing experience that he never forgets and which will be useful to him, whatever his subsequent occupation.

Experience in the teaching of general practice likewise presents two extremes. At one end lies the academic department which conceives its function to be lecturing the students about the problems of general practice, the range of patients seen there, and the organization of health centres. In many instances these are augmented by large classes of students attending sessions in a university general practice. The most effective scheme seems to be one in which the student participates actively. It is an advantage for general practice to be a part of the Department of Community Medicine so that it is seen as a part of the service to the community and particularly as part of the NHS. Sessions in which problems of specific patients seen in general practice are considered by general practitioners, hospital doctors, and social service workers form an admirable introduction to the NHS as a whole. In some medical schools, for example Newcastle, Nottingham, and Southampton, the student is introduced by a general practitioner to patients in the first week or month at the medical school. At Newcastle, for example, he meets a pregnant woman, follows her to delivery and sees both mother and child during the next few years. He keeps a record of the development of the child, for example when it smiles for the first time. He is also introduced to a problem family so that he becomes interested in behavioural and community aspects of medicine. Students greatly appreciate presenting one of their cases before their colleagues and the teachers whose specialty is relevant and the subsequent opportunities for discussion. Another device greatly appreciated by students is to live in with the general practitioner and to do everything that he does, including night visits. This, however, makes such demands on the household and particularly the doctor's wife that it is rarely possible these days.

In general it has to be said that the successful teaching of these subjects depends on two things. First, the extent to which the student actively participates and, second, the extent to which medical and community aspects are emphasized and illustrated by work in the field rather than in the lecture theatre.

Academic departments of general practice have, I think, proved their worth in the university medical school. Their worth is not to teach students in university departments of general practice but to organize and arrange such teaching and the early contact between students and patients. If the student is to understand the problems of general practice he should see them in a typical NHS practice. The professor will recruit enough local practitioners of sufficient calibre and enthusiasm to ensure that students can be allocated in pairs for practical training. In general these practitioners are paid much less than they would be for training postgraduates. However, a university title in many cases is sufficient compensation.

5

Examinations

Examinations would become the master and not the servant
of Higher Education.   *Lord Haldane* (23)

The identification of examinations with education was a
contentious misconception in English education.
                                        Lord Haldane (23)

It is one of the dangers of any system of examination that
we may come to value only what we can test.
                        Science Masters Association (24)

These warnings cannot be too often repeated to medical educators
of today, for they emphasize what has actually happened.

Examinations naturally loom large in medical education. In
fact they tend to dominate it so far as both the pupil and the
teacher are concerned. This is not hard to understand. The Medical Acts have made it imperative for the licensing bodies and the
General Medical Council to ascertain that the candidate has sufficient knowledge to practise efficiently in medicine, surgery, and
midwifery. Until now, no method has been discovered to ensure
this, other than the formal examination. Even for the certification
of the specialist, the formal examination is an integral part of the
process, though the Todd Commission emphasized that this
should not be so. Moreover, as we have seen, the laudable object
of monitoring the student's progress by continuous assessment
has degenerated into frequent examination.

Examinations as they now exist in the medical curriculum are
designed almost solely for testing what is called factual knowledge: though a little thought shows that it is nothing of the
kind, it is the testing of the prevailing dogmas accepted by the
examiners. The preferred medium is the multiple choice question
or MCQ in which the candidate is asked a question and required
to select one or more of, say, five possible answers as being the
correct one. As in this example:

Compared with young adults, healthy *children* tend to have a

(*a*) higher plasma inorganic phosphorus concentration

(*b*) higher serum calcium concentration

(*c*) higher alkaline phosphatase activity in serum

(*d*) lower whole blood haemoglobin level

(*e*) higher serum Ig A concentration.

This is, of course, a good question but hardly the basis on which one would choose a doctor for one's children.

The advantages of such questions are that the form on which the candidate enters his answers can be marked mechanically, and the results can be put through a computer and analysed for replicability and discriminating power. The difference between good MCQs and the rest is of the same order as the difference between a virtuoso pianist and the ordinary family performer. Anderson's book contains good examples (25). Nearly all examining bodies keep a bank of MCQs which they guard carefully. Fortunately, setting the questions involves a great deal of time and trouble, but all the marking is done by machines and their operators.

Most students like MCQs and the GMC does not disapprove. Nevertheless, it is generally admitted that MCQs have these disadvantages:

1. They are artificial. In real life factual recall is not aided by, say, five possible choices—the range of choice is infinite. Therefore successful completion of MCQ depends on technique. It is a game which some students master easily, others with difficulty. Some of the best students find them difficult. It is possible to know too much.

2. They often concentrate on trivialities. To increase their difficulty, the examiners must seek for uncommon knowledge.

3. The solutions are not strictly factual: they represent opinions. They are objective only in the sense that the answers have been agreed by the examiners.

4. They do not test the following important educational objectives:

(*a*) the candidate's ability to express himself concisely, lucidly, and grammatically;

(b) his capacity for having original ideas;

(c) his ability to gather and set out evidence, assess its validity, and form a judgement.

MCQs demand an answer without the evidence on which that answer is based. They remind me of the trial scene in Alice:

> 'Let the jury consider their verdict,' the King said, for about the twentieth time that day.
> 'No, no!' said the Queen, 'Sentence first—verdict afterwards.'

As a method of assessing competence, which is what they seek to do, MCQs are also fallacious. The competence they assess is the competence for remembering and reproducing what they were taught. But that is not what makes a competent physician or surgeon. To illustrate my point, let me quote an instance. My best friend, L. R. Wager, failed his medical test for the 1932 Everest expedition. He could not hold his breath long enough, and he could not blow up a column of mercury high enough. These tests had been developed and evaluated for high altitude flying during the First World War. Like the MCQs they were quantitative and replicable. Therefore Wager was judged unsuited for climbing at high altitudes. But as he was a very competent and experienced mountaineer they took him on the expedition to back up the men who were more promising. Alas, when they got well up the mountain, the men who had done well in the tests developed Cheyne Stokes respiration which prevented them from sleeping, or they developed breathlessness and palpitations, and they had to be sent down. Wager, on the other hand, plodded on and acclimatized so well that he was chosen for the first assault party, and is one of the select few who have climbed at 28,000 ft without oxygen. Thus the test, though replicable and quantitative, did not test the point at issue. Similarly, MCQs, though replicable and quantitative, do not necessarily test the kind of knowledge that is useful to the doctor and they certainly make no claim to test the other capabilities that he needs.

An extension of the MCQ to allow it to test solutions to a more complicated problem has also been devised and developed in the US and UK (see Fleming *et al.*, 1976 [26]). Applied to medicine the candidate is given a few facts about a patient or a fairly full

case report and asked a succession of questions which again he has
to declare as true or false. Two examples given to prospective candidates in a medical school I visited are :

1. You are called to see an elderly patient who has recently
been admitted with haematemesis and melaena. Name three
diseases, other than peptic ulcer, which could be responsible.

(Typically acceptable answers would include gastric cancer,
oesophageal varices, oesophageal mucosal tear.)

2. Give three important features of the early management
of acute gastrointestinal bleeding. (Acceptable answers include 'Estimate degree of blood loss clinically' [or variants on
this theme]; 'measure haemoglobin'; 'take blood for group
and cross match'; 'consider informing surgeon of potential
problem if rebleeding occurs'.)

These two examples expose the fallacies of this and similar examinations. In my fifty years of clinical experience I have never
seen a patient admitted for a haematemasis because of an oesophageal tear, though I myself have twice had blood in the vomit
after repeated and severe emesis. On the other hand, I had many
patients who had ingested aspirin tablets, thus producing a gastric
erosion. Indomethazine can do the same. (When I wrote this, I
was relying on the memory of my own unanalysed experience.
Since then Allan and Dykes [27] [1976] have analysed 300 patients admitted to the Birmingham General Hospital for gastrointestinal haemorrhage. 147 had peptic ulcer, 51 had gastric
erosions, 15 had gastric cancer, 12 hiatus hernia, 6 had oesophageal varices, and 6 the Mallory-Weiss syndrome [of oesophageal tear]; the remainder were miscellaneous or uncertain.)
Again, in answer to the second question, I would rate a half-
hourly blood pressure chart as the most important, since a fall of
pressure is the first indication of a renewed haemorrhage, the com-
monest cause of death.

The point is that these so-called objective tests are only objective because the examiners are agreed on which answers are
correct and which not. The method and the trust which the contemporary medical hierarchy places on it represent to me a ter-
rifying return to authoritarianism and the tyranny of dogma. Is
history going to repeat itself? And are we on the threshold of an-

other Dark Age? This then is the current trend in the form of
examinations in medicine. And I cannot, and would not wish to,
disguise that I think it a most unfortunate trend.

The increasing use of the MCQ is due to the shortcomings of
the older type of so-called essay question commonly used in medical examinations until recently. An example would be—'Describe the symptoms, signs, and treatment of ulcerative colitis.'
Now this is a very clumsy method of asking the candidate to
dredge up from his memory the appropriate pages from his
favourite textbook or his lecture notes. The candidate could be
forgiven for shortening his answer into lists and for omitting to
write a single grammatical sentence. It saved time, and his examiner rather liked it, because it saved his time too. The competence it tests is broadly the same as that of the MCQ. Moreover,
Bull (1956)(28) showed that the errors in marking this type of
question, between different examiners marking the same answer,
and between a single examiner marking the answer on different
occasions, was so large as to suggest their very dubious validity.
The demise of this type of question is, in every way, a blessing
to medicine, to students, to teachers, and indeed to intellectual in-
tegrity.

MCQs are designed for the convenience of the examiners.
Once the questions are decided the examiner has little more to do
than scrutinize the marks supplied by the computer and decide
the levels for pass and for fail. MCQs are probably irreplaceable
for examinations like the MRCP and for two reasons. They enable large numbers to be examined (600 candidates in the MRCP)
and they are demonstrably fair and free of personal bias. This
is important when the candidates come not only from many
schools but from several different countries. These considerations do not, however, apply so much to university examinations,
especially to class examinations that so often masquerade as continuous assessment. The proper place of the MCQ is undoubtedly
to discard candidates who clearly fail. If they are used in examinations like the MRCP they should be supplemented by other
questions which test the candidate's ability to display evidence,
to argue from it, and to convey ideas and information lucidly,
concisely, and grammatically. Thus the MRCP tries to test the
candidate's fitness to hold a post as a specialist physician. It is
not enough that he should be able to make the right diagnosis

and to suggest the appropriate further steps to be taken and the treatment to be given; unless he can set this out lucidly and grammatically in the letter he writes to the general practitioner he is incompetent. At present there is no test of this competence.

In the MRCP it would be logical to ask the candidate to write a letter to the patient's doctor about the subject of his long case. A satisfactory letter would be a condition for passing the examination, as it should be, if its purpose is to test competence to act as a consultant physician.

My main objection to MCQs is that they have come to dominate and even to monopolize examinations in Medicine. They have their place, but it is a restricted place.

Unfortunately, medicine is still intellectually isolated. Few people are aware of a new approach, conceived some thirty years ago by the Science Masters(24) amongst others (Appendix IV). In 1950 they pointed out that teachers tried to teach their pupils two things: first facts, and second how to arrange and interpret facts. They suggested that there should be two types of question: first a test of knowledge, including facts, definitions, and principles; second, a paper that would test the ability of the candidate to use knowledge, for example to marshal the points of an argument in orderly sequence or to write out clear instructions for the performance of an experiment. They said

> It should be remembered that an important part of the training we try to give to our pupils lies in the ability to express themselves with clarity in English and in this type of question candidates who have not acquired this skill are automatically penalized.

While these principles and methods were explored by science masters they had little impact on medicine. We introduced them in medicine in the Final MB at Manchester and they were introduced into the Final BM at Oxford. A paper for surgery is an example given in Appendix V. Unfortunately, neither I nor any of my colleagues tested these examination techniques for replicability and discriminating power as Fleming and others (1976)(26) have done for MCQs. Thus the experiment came to a halt.

The most telling criticism of the present form of examinations in medicine is that it neglects entirely their educational function. The questions asked in examinations are by far the most sure indication that the pupil receives from his teachers as to what is important and what is unimportant. His teachers may deliver long and repeated diatribes and they may exhort this and that, but if these important attainments are not part of the tests by which the pupil's adequacy is judged, then what is the function of these tests? It is understandable if today's student considers that because many universities and the Royal College of Physicians judge his competence without testing his ability to display and marshal evidence and form a judgement and to convey information and opinions clearly and succinctly in writing and speech, therefore these attainments are unimportant. A decline in literacy and in scholarship must follow as the night the day.

I would judge that one of the most important tasks awaiting medical educators is the development and testing of techniques for examining for factual knowledge on the one hand and, on the other, for the capacity to arrange and assess evidence and to convey information and ideas concisely and precisely in writing and speech. Granted that MCQs have a dubious basis of reliability, because what is reliable is merely the prearranged opinion of the examiners, I feel confident that a better alternative would emerge. The Merrison Committee (11) recommended that the GMC should undertake or commission research into medical education. I can think of nothing that is more urgently needed than an enquiry into the educational value and reliability of different types of examination in the field of medicine.

I would like to close this section by quoting the General Medical Council's Recommendations of 1967 (10):

> 1. In reducing the load of the all-embracing final examination, it is important to avoid the hazard of burdening the student with excessive and too frequent assessments. There may be a risk that in these matters of assessing and testing students a teacher will 'see and approve the better but follow the worse course'.

> 2. The examination system designed by the University should aim at contributing to the education of the student. The primary object should be to test (and in doing so to foster) the student's understanding of what he has learnt and his capacity for thinking for himself, and not simply his factual knowledge.

6

The special case of London

Medical education in London presents a special case of great importance. At the time of the Royal Commission(5) one half of those who graduated in medicine at British universities were taught in London. About 60 per cent of all postgraduate students in British Faculties of Medicine were to be found in London. Moreover, in London there is only one university which is federal and contains 15 medical schools of which 12 are undergraduate and 3 postgraduate. The latter comprise the London School of Hygiene and Tropical Medicine, the Royal Postgraduate Medical School, and the British Postgraduate Medical Federation which comprises 13 postgraduate specialist medical institutes. The arrangements in London received special consideration by both the Goodenough and Todd Committees. My treatment will be brief.

Postgraduate education

The British Postgraduate Medical Federation and the special postgraduate institutes have been the subject of numerous reports, one of which was chaired by myself (30). The position of the Royal Postgraduate Medical School is no longer controversial. It serves an established purpose in the particular field of training an élite who will occupy positions of importance in the worlds of medical education and research in this country and abroad.

The position of the specialist postgraduate institutes is less assured. Several of them have achieved world-wide renown and positions of eminence so they are likely to continue indefinitely and in association with their specialist hospitals. The fate of the others is less certain and I shall say nothing about them.

The Postgraduate Medical Federation and its central office is essential to the functioning of the whole. There was a time when, apart from the very much smaller Edinburgh centre, it was virtually the only place to which a student from outside London,

including foreign countries and those of the British Common-
wealth applied for advanced clinical training. Now much of its
advisory function is being taken over by the Central Council but
it supervises postgraduate education in the four metropolitan
regions. It brings together the special postgraduate institutes and
it arranges courses on special advanced subjects which are attended by audiences widely drawn from London and the provinces.

Postgraduate medical education through district general hospitals and postgraduate medical centres is organized into four
regions, each of which has its postgraduate dean. The regions
are North-East, North-West, South-East, and South-West. The
number of postgraduate medical centres in the session 1974–5
were respectively 23, 18, 17, and 15.

The reorganization of local government and of the NHS has
dealt unkindly with these arrangements. During the Second
World War, London and its environs were organized on a sector
basis such that each sector had a teaching hospital which was
responsible for staffing. Now the London teaching hospitals are
in districts which are separated from the rest of the region and
with which communication has become so cumbrous as to be
virtually nonexistent. Thus, unlike Southampton or Birmingham,
the teaching hospitals do not have a large sphere of influence that
they can call their own. This is the major difference between
postgraduate medical education in the London region and the rest
of the country, and it is greatly to London's disadvantage.

Undergraduate education

The Todd Commission recommended that the twelve medical
schools in London should be reduced to six and each twin become
part of a multifaculty institution. Their reasons were:

1. The undesirable concentration of medical students in London. 'The London medical schools teach nearly one half of those
who graduate in medicine at British universities.'

2. The medical schools had been dominated by their hospitals
and by the Royal Colleges rather than by the University which
came later.

3. Medical education should take place in a multifaculty in-
stution. Medical students should mingle with other students.

They stressed 'the need for close contact between the medical, natural and social sciences at the teaching and research level'. 'Medical schools cannot hope to offer separately from their own resources adequate teaching in the range of options we believe will be desirable.'

4. They thought the medical schools were too small, and had great difficulty 'in attracting financial support comparable with that made available to medical schools in other British centres'.

> The twelve London undergraduate schools at present have an incomplete and uneven range of clinical Chairs. They are notably deficient in chairs of Obstetrics and Gynaecology, Paediatrics, Psychiatry and Social Medicine. The resulting disability suffered by medical education in London will become increasingly grave as teaching in the medical curriculum grows more dependent on the services of highly trained special staff, on modern expensive equipment, and on the associated research activities.

They therefore recommended that the twelve undergraduate schools be reduced to six by combination according to the following scheme:

(*a*) St Bartholomew's Hospital Medical College with the London Hospital Medical College.

(*b*) University College Hospital Medical School with the Royal Free Hospital.

(*c*) St Mary's Hospital Medical School with the Middlesex Hospital Medical School.

(*d*) Guy's Hospital Medical School with King's College Hospital Medical School.

(*e*) Westminster Medical School with Charing Cross Hospital Medical School (the rebuilding of the latter at Fulham is planned).

(*f*) St Thomas's Hospital Medical School with St George's Hospital Medical School (the rebuilding of the latter at Tooting is planned).

They considered that it would be possible for the twins to join with another institution of the University and become a multi-faculty institution. Thus the St Bartholomew's–London would move to a site near Queen Mary College. The University College–Royal Free combination would have its preclinical department at University College. The Middlesex–Mary's combination would become the medical faculty of Bedford College. Guys–KCH would be integrated in time with King's College. Westminster–Charing Cross combination would become the medical faculty of Imperial College. St George's and St Thomas's combination would become in course of time the medical faculty of a new multifaculty institution developing out of the Chelsea College of Science and Technology.

The Todd proposals unfortunately neglected geography. If we take, for example, the St Mary's–Middlesex–Bedford College group, we may ask where the giant multifaculty institution would be sited? On the Middlesex Hospital site which, being close to Oxford Street, has some of the most expensive property in London and is away from the main centres of population? On the St Mary's site, equally congested unless there was an extensive destruction of Paddington Station or of residential property nearby? Or at Bedford College—and how would Londoners feel about the destruction of Regent's Park? Even trying to make them work together, as they now do, has insuperable difficulties. It took me forty-five minutes to get from St Mary's to the Middlesex by public transport. In a car the time is reduced to twenty minutes, provided the car can be parked at either end as is the case with the Dean—but with no-one else. Moreover, as universities increase in size it becomes progressively more difficult to house everything on the same site. Hence the medical school at Birmingham is more than a quarter of a mile from the other faculties and Aberdeen still further. The Welsh National School of Medicine is about half an hour from University College, Cardiff. Moreover, their statements that the London schools were too small to enable them to attract adequate staff are just not true. At the time of my survey, St Mary's had four Fellows of the Royal Society and the Middlesex two. The provincial schools outside Oxford and Cambridge which I visited often had none and never more than two.

The detailed Todd proposals would not have been expected to fare well, nor have they. St Mary's and the Middlesex set up a joint Committee which still meets. They have a few joint appointments with Bedford. But the facts of geography are insuperable. The Guy's–King's, Westminster–Charing Cross, and St Thomas's–St George's never made any progress. Charing Cross and St George's, both rebuilt on new sites are going it alone. St

Thomas's, Westminster, and King's College had a prolonged flirtation, but geography is too strong.

More successful seemed to be the Bart's–London–Queen Mary College enterprise. The three institutions collaborated with enthusiasm and good will. A site on a former Jewish cemetery was obtained next to Queen Mary College to house a preclinical school. Several joint appointments were made. But the distance between Queen Mary College and the London Hospital is such that it takes thirty to forty minutes by foot or public transport; the time taken to St Bartholomew's is even longer. The development of this scheme is indefinitely postponed for lack of money.

The most promising seemed to be the UC–UCH–Royal Free combination. University College planned to develop to house within its boundaries an enlarged preclinical school which would provide for both clinical schools. Consequently, provision for the preclinical departments in the new Royal Free Medical School at Hampstead was stopped and the medical school built without them. The departments at University College are halted indefinitely for lack of money. The Royal Free limps along with its old overcrowded preclinical school at Hunter Street.

I am doubtful whether even the Royal Free–UC venture could have been a success. I spent nine years at UCH, and was one of the few members of the staff who collaborated with my colleagues across the road. But access was easy because of propinquity and an underground passage. A much bigger school and its development on another part of the site would have made contact much more difficult. There were no advantages for the Royal Free other than contact between their preclinical students and those of other faculties. The Royal Free would have had a preclinical school that was an appendage to a large institution whose clinical contacts would be with its rival UCH. As it is, the implementation of Todd for the Royal Free has been little short of a disaster.

In general the decision to implement the Todd Report so far as London was concerned has done nothing except to delay desirable developments in the London schools and cause frustration and waste of time to the staff who tried to implement them. There is a very strong case for trying to reorganize university education in London on the basis of a number of multifaculty institutions, each with a faculty of medicine and teaching hospital. But this was not the way to do it.

In comparison with the provinces London faces an enormous disadvantage in not having its own region in which to forge links between the medical school, the teaching hospital, the district general hospitals, and the local community services.

In my view an opportunity to develop undergraduate and postgraduate education together by restarting the wartime sectors was tragically missed. The reorganization of the NHS has now made it virtually impossible.

7

Conclusions

The pace of medical advance, both scientific and technological, is now so fast that it is essential for every doctor to be able to continue to educate himself till he ceases to practice medicine. With the growth of postgraduate medical institutes since 1961 the physical means to do this are now available throughout the country, with few exceptions. The outstanding task today is therefore to ensure that the appetite for, and habits of, self education are developed and acquired during the formal processes of education. Long-established educational theory and practice suggests that this should be effected early in the educational process, that is during the undergraduate period.

Graduate or postgraduate education for the specialties

The arrangements throughout the country are now, or shortly will be, adequate to offer the young medical graduate opportunities to be trained in the knowledge, techniques, and attitudes necessary for the efficient practice of any specialty, including that of general practice. It is the intention that the new National Health Service (Vocational Training) Act of 1976 will require that, after the appointed day, the Medical Practices Committee shall refuse any application by a medical practitioner for the provision of general medical services unless he has acquired 'prescribed experience'. Prescribed experience has yet to be defined.

The Joint Committees on Higher Medical, Surgical, and Psychiatric Training have organized courses in each region that train for each specialty and its examination requirements. The courses, and those who attend them, are inevitably examination oriented. Day release enables, with varying efficiency, would be practitioners to attend courses. The chief hindrances are distance and the pressure of NHS work on both trainers and trainees.

The most important part of graduate education is 'in service' training through the carrying out of jobs of increasing responsibility.

1. The first two posts are those prescribed by Act of Parliament for full registration, the so-called pre-registration house appointments. The universities are responsible for approving these posts, a process now being carried out with greater efficiency by the regional postgraduate committees.

2. Succeeding posts are posts of increasing responsibility through senior house officer, registrar, and senior registrar grades.

The number and distribution of these posts still poses problems which are beyond the scope of this report. The inspection and approval for training purposes has been largely carried out by the relevant joint committees. This process has been cumbrous, enormously expensive, particularly in terms of skilled medical manpower, and has tended to become rather rigid. It is the expectation and hope that experience will enable a less expensive and more flexible system to be devised.

The duration of these training posts is considerably longer than that required for similar experience in North America and the continent of Europe.

Each of the specialties employs examinations as a part of the process of approval for specialist practice. These examinations in general are tending to have a negative educational value. They are becoming increasingly of the so-called 'objective' type in which the candidate is rewarded for repeating dogmas approved by the examiners. In some specialties, for example, medicine, there is no longer any test of literacy or scholarship. Some specialties, notably obstetrics and community medicine, still require the submission of original written work with appropriate references to the literature.

The applicants for the different specialties are unequally distributed. The steps taken to inform senior students and young graduates about career prospects in the specialties are quite inadequate.

Undergraduate education

1. Applicants for university places choose medicine more frequently than any other discipline. Medical students are thus amongst the ablest of their generation.

2. The training of medical students in the undergraduate period has in the past failed as an education because attempts have been made to ensure that the student on graduation is fit to practice efficiently every kind of medical specialty. This has never been a realistic idea within living memory. It is still less so today. The doctor who considers himself adequate to practise every specialty is a public menace.

3. The arrangements and facilities now provided and being provided for graduate education offer adequate training for the practice of each specialty, including general practice. The undergraduate period is therefore freed for its proper function, namely the training of the student's mind as an instrument of inquiry, precision, and judgement in the context of man, society, and disease. This survey has shown that this objective is only attained by a minority of medical graduates. The chief causes for this failure are too many subjects, too many lectures, and the development of the so-called objective methods of examination, multiple choice questions and their variations, whose defects have been noted.

4. There are now some thirty subjects, each presided over by a university professor, which form the basis of the medical curriculum. Attempts have been made to lessen the burden on the student by the following methods.

(*a*) Integration between disciplines.

(*b*) Continuous assessment rather than a few massive examinations.

(*c*) Small group teaching.

5. At too many schools the undergraduates complain that they are bored, that they are treated as data banks, that they are expected to listen to lectures, memorize them and reproduce them for examination purposes, that independent intellectual effort is discouraged because there is no time and it does not count for assessment. This survey suggests that these complaints are justified.

6. Integrated teaching has been developed in many schools. In very few schools all the subjects taught are included in an integrated curriculum. In most other schools an attempt is made at integration but some subjects have remained aloof. Integration

eases the task of the student but increases the burden on the teacher. He has to teach when asked and not at set times and has to take cognizance of what his colleagues in different disciplines are teaching.

7. Very few schools and very few subjects have found it possible to assess students on the quality of the work that they actually do during their courses. Most rely on repeated small examinations. Increasingly these are of the multiple choice type.

8. The purpose of small group teaching is to encourage a dialogue between teachers and taught, to encourage students to work up subjects and present the answers for criticism. Far too often they are ill-prepared mini-lectures or cram classes, frankly designed to answer examination questions.

9. In a few schools all students are required at some time in their course to write a thesis based on an inquiry conducted by the student himself. These students have to use the library and quote references correctly. In some schools this does not happen and students graduate without ever having learned to use a library or had any test of the ability to write or speak lucidly, concisely, and grammatically.

10. A few schools require every student to study about a year in depth. Southampton is the only school which succeeds in fitting this into the five-year curriculum. It is thus a most interesting and important experiment.

11. Every school provides an opportunity for some students to spend an extra year studying one subject in depth: the Honours year. In Oxford and Nottingham all students do this. Students who have been fortunate enough to undergo this experience are truly educated in that they know how to set about asking a question, providing evidence to answer it, judging the validity of that evidence and setting out the evidence and the conclusions based on it lucidly and concisely. These students are educated and fit to embrace the opportunities provided by graduate and continuing education.

12. The value or otherwise of a medical education depends more perhaps on the attitude of mind of the teachers than on the details of the curriculum. Teachers who regard the student as a

passive object to whom information is to be fed and regurgitated on demand tend to produce less lively young people than those who regard the student as a person in whom interest can be aroused and who can learn to discover things for himself. Kindling the flame is more rewarding than filling the pot.

13. Many of the defects of medical education can be attributed to examinations. Multiple choice questions and their variants are replicable and can discriminate. But, though they are alleged to test knowledge of fact, what they test is knowledge of current dogma. An outstanding need is to introduce and test examinations which test

(*a*) The candidate's knowledge of fact.

(*b*) His capacity to display evidence, assess its validity, and argue from it.

(*c*) His capacity to express himself lucidly, precisely, and concisely.

14. Looking back over the whole of my survey I am alarmed by the efficiency of the bureaucratic control, which tends to constrain the medical student of today. In the undergraduate period he is tyrannized by the frequent examinations of continuous assessment. In the graduate period he has to fit into the mould being fashioned by the Joint Committees on Higher Specialist Training. Will medicine in the future produce any scientist of distinction or innovators of any kind?

Final comment

Having finished the parts, I can now survey the whole. The following points stand out.

1. No single body, be it university or GMC, has hitherto considered medical education as a whole. It is high time that this was done. To my mind, it would be a public service if the GMC accepted responsibility for the whole of medical education, undergraduate and postgraduate (graduate). It is to be hoped that its recommendations will continue to be as enlightened as those of 1967.

2. I have become deeply concerned at the growing regimentation of the doctor in training. In the undergraduate period his in-

tellectual freedom is seriously curtailed by the tyranny of frequently repeated examinations, most in the guise of continuous assessment. This tyranny is compounded by the move towards multiple choice questions which, though at their best valid tests of a certain kind of knowledge, encourage the student to learn answers without the evidence on which they are based, and thus encourage bad intellectual habits and discourage literacy. In the graduate period, the rigorous system of job succession and job approval, being imposed by the Joint Committees on Higher Medical and Surgical Training, will take most of the adventure out of that period, and make the lot of the young scientist intolerable.

We are, I think, in danger of putting the medical student and the young doctor in a straitjacket that we are now fashioning. We are making the fit very tight. This is being done in the cause of eliminating bad doctors. I fear that it will also eliminate the best, particularly the creative minds, on whom future developments will depend. This is an issue of such gravity that I find it difficult to stress it sufficiently. It is particularly unfortunate coming at a time when medical students are better than they have ever been before.

APPENDICES

APPENDIX I

Institutions visited in the course of preparing this report

The medical schools visited were those of Birmingham, Cambridge, Glasgow, Manchester, Newcastle, Nottingham, Oxford, St Andrews, Southampton Universities, and the University of Wales, and Middlesex Hospital, St Mary's Hospital, St Thomas's Hospital Medical Schools in the University of London. At most of these medical schools I was accompanied by my wife who took most excellent notes.

Each school provided me with the appropriate documents concerning staff, students, history, the curriculum, and their plans for the future. In many instances these took the form of memoranda already supplied to the University Grants Committee. We spent a minimum of two days and a maximum of five days at each of these schools visiting the preclinical departments, the clinical departments, including the hospitals, and at least one postgraduate institution in the region. We usually saw the Vice-Chancellor, the Dean and his staff, the Professors or their representatives, the junior staff of the pre-clinical departments, the junior staff of the clinical departments, the NHS consultants, the NHS junior staff, the students, and the Postgraduate Dean with his regional officers and Postgraduate Committee. In each of these universities, we were hospitably entertained, often by the Vice-Chancellor himself or herself. The Nuffield Provincial Hospitals Trust also enabled us to entertain some of our hosts. It is a great pleasure to express our deep appreciation for their courtesy and hospitality and for giving us so much of their valuable time.

In addition we paid shorter visits, often informally, to the following universities and medical schools: Edinburgh University, Leicester University, Charing Cross Medical School, the Royal Free Hospital Medical School, and University College, London.

The Presidents and senior officers of the following Royal Colleges and Faculties in London kindly arranged for me to visit them, often entertaining me to lunch to discuss their plans for the conduct and supervision of postgraduate education in their specialty: the Faculty of Anaesthetists, the Faculty of Community Medicine, Royal College of Obstetricians and Gynaecologists, the Royal College of Pathologists, the Royal College of Physicians, the Royal College of Psychiatrists, the Royal College of Surgeons, the Faculty of Radiologists, and the Royal College of General Practitioners. I had several discussions with the officers of the Central Council for Postgraduate Education in England and Wales and some with the Central Council for Postgraduate Education in Scotland (mostly by telephone). In London I did not visit the schools of the Postgraduate Medical Federation but I paid several visits to the Director of the British Postgraduate Medical Federation and his staff at their central office. In addition to the Postgraduate Medical Centres that I visited as part of my university visits, I also visited the following: Canterbury, Chelmsford, Hastings, Northampton, Norwich, and Windsor. I was privileged to chair a conference on vocational training for general practice at Taunton.

APPENDIX II

Programme for the month of February for the Postgraduate Medical Institute, Stoke on Trent

B.M.A.

Wed.	23rd	8.15 p.m.	"Aspects of the Management of Angina" - Dr.E.G.Wade. Consultant Cardiologist, Manchester.

B.M.A. LADIES

Wed.	23rd	2.30 p.m.

BRITISH HEART FOUNDATION

Thur.	10th	5.00 p.m.	"Sudden Coronary Death" Professor D.G.Julian.

ROYAL COLLEGE OF NURSING

Thur.	17th	7.30 p.m. Annual General Meeting

N.S.PHARMACEUTICAL SOCIETY

Tue.	8th	8.00 p.m.	"Pharmacy in America and Great Britain". -Professor A.H. Beckett.

N.S.DENTAL SURGEONS

Tue.	8th	8.00 p.m.

BRITISH OPTICAL ASSOCIATION

Wed.	9th	8.00 p.m.

STAFFS. OCCUPATIONAL HEALTH

Wed.	16th	7.30 p.m.

SOCIETY OF CHIROPODISTS

Thur.	24th	7.00 p.m.

SECTION OF PSYCHIATRY

Fri.	25th	8.00 p.m.	Dr. Julian Bird.

WEEKLY SEMINAR

Mon.	7th	5.00 p.m.	"Exercise after Myocardial Infarction" -Dr.P.Carson.
	14th	5.00 p.m.	"Some Aspects of Geriatric Medicine" - Dr.W.F.Rogers.
	21st	5.00 p.m.	"Sero-Negative Spond-Arthritis" Dr.T.E.Hothersall.
	28th	5.00 p.m.	"Pituitary Function Tests" - Dr. W.Van't Hoff.

ORTHOPAEDIC POST-GRADUATE

Wed.	2nd	5.30 p.m.	X-Ray Conference
	9th	5.30 p.m.	Journal Club
	16th	5.30 p.m.	Symposium.
	23rd	5.30 p.m.	"Isotope Scanning in Relation to Orthopaedic & Trauma Surgery". Dr. M.Venkateswaran.

MEDICAL STAFF ROUND

Tue.	1st, 8th, 15th & 22nd at 12.00 Noon

SKIN DEPARTMENT

Tue.	1st	1.00 p.m.	Journal Club (Consultants)
	8th	1.00 p.m.	"Lichenoid Reactions" Dr.E.M.Donaldson.
	15th	1.00 p.m.	Journal Club (Junior Staff)
	22nd	1.00 p.m.	"Bullous Eruptions" - Dr. R.Summerly

G.P.JOURNAL CLUB

Wed.	2nd	12.45p.m.	"Natural History and the Incidence of Angina and Infarction in General Practice".

G.P. TRAINERS WORKSHOP

Wed.	2nd	8.00 p.m.

G.P. TRAINEES MEETINGS

Thur.	3rd	2.00 p.m.	"General Practitioner Terms of Service" - Dr.M.T.Sweetno
	10th	2.00 p.m.	"Appointments Systems" - Dr. P. Exon.
Tur.	17th	2.00 p.m.	"The Doctor & Industry" - Dr.E.G.Hughes.
	24th	2.00 p.m.	"Fertility Problems" - Mr.M.R.Glass & Dr.H,W.Thos

CLINICAL/SURGICAL MEETINGS

Mon.	7th, 14th, 21st & 28th at 5.30 p.m.

G.P. LUNCHTIME MEETING

Wed.	9th	12.30 p.m.	"Recent Advances in Oncology Dr. R. Lindup.

RESEARCH CLUB

Sat.	12th & 26th at 11.00 a.m.

BIOCHEMICAL MEETING

Wed.	16th	12.00 Noon

RADIOLOGY LECTURE

Wed.	16th	5.15 p.m.

PERIDONTOLOGY POST-GRADUATE

Fri.	18th	2.00 p.m.	Course
Sat.	19th	9.00 a.m. - 6.00 p.m.	Course.

COMMITTEE MEETINGS

Wed.	2nd	3.30 p.m.	Radiologists Sub-Committee.
		7.45 p.m.	Cystic Fibrosis Committee.
Tue.	8th	5.00 p.m.	Medical Advisory Committee.
Mon.	14th	5.00 p.m.	Psychiatric Specialists' Sub-Committee.
Tue.	22nd	5.00 a.m.	Surgical Specialists' Sub-Committee.
Mon.	28th	5.30 p.m.	Anaesthetic Advisory Sub-Committee.

DENTAL SURGERY ASSISTANTS

| Mon. | 21st | 7.45 p.m. | "Aspects of Speech Therapy". |

NEUROPATHOLOGY MEETING

| Wed. | 23rd | 12.00 Noon |

ADVANCED NOTICE

Thursday 3rd March 5.30 p.m. WADE LECTURE - "Breast Cancer - A Tale of Three Women" Professor A.P.M. Forrest.

Sat. 26th March 9 a.m. Section of General Practice. SYMPOSIUM.
- 6 p.m.

Please note that there will not be a Dental Lunchtime Meeting on Tuesday, 15th February 1977.

APPENDIX III

Report on the Southampton Medical School

The boldest and in many ways the most successful new curriculum is that of the University of Southampton. It owes much to the pioneering work of Newcastle. Preclinical, clinical, and social sciences are closely integrated and it succeeds in incorporating what is in effect an honours year into its five-year curriculum. Moreover it succeeds in introducing students to patients early in the course in a way that they can understand without a detailed knowledge of medical sciences. A unique feature of the Southampton school is that it was conceived jointly by the university and the local regional authority in the National Health Service (at that time the Wessex Regional Hospital Board). It sees itself as an organization centred on a university but not confined to it, bringing in many disciplines and professions, intimately concerned with the prevention and treatment of illness, and acting as a centre of academic resources for the health services throughout the region.

The first three years of the curriculum includes not only the basic course work in the biological and social sciences, including pathology, but also a substantial amount of contact with patients and instruction in clinical techniques. Three features are sufficiently novel to be noteworthy. The first is that almost all of the physiological teaching and some of the anatomy, pathology, pharmacology, and epidemiology is presented in the form of a series of systems courses, nine in all, starting with the reproductive system and followed by the cardiovascular system, respiratory system, etc. Despite the obvious practical difficulty of achieving integration and avoiding unnecessary overlap and repetition in a multidisciplinary approach, the systems courses are proving popular and there is a demand from the students for further material to be incorporated in them—for instance, from biochemistry. Once it had been decided that some special pathology should be incorporated in the systems course general pathology and microbiology had to be introduced very early—namely, in the first year. This has worked well.

A second noteworthy feature of the first three years is the gradual introduction of the student to the patient from the beginning of the course. In the first year each student meets patients in their homes with the family doctor and, in parallel with the human reproduction course, follows a patient through the ante-natal clinic and attends her delivery and post-natal examination. By the sixth term the student is beginning to learn the basic techniques of history-taking and examination, and in the third year he spends more than half his time in clinical work in medicine, surgery, obstetrics and gynaecology, geriatric medicine, psychiatry, and child health. The assumption on which this approach is based is that there is an almost universal desire on the part of medical students to have contact with patients, and that by encouraging this from the beginning one sustains and develops their drive to study. A second expected benefit of the gradual introduction of clinical work is that the students will earlier acquire skill in communicating with a wide range of people and will come to the bedside for their formal instruction in the third year with a good deal more confidence than their predecessors. On the debit side there is a risk that his contact with patients will distract the student from a proper study of the essential basic sciences.

Another feature of this part of the curriculum which deserves emphasis is the teaching in primary medical care in the third year. They believe that the simplest way to learn about the practice of medicine outside the hospital is to see and participate in it, and that this is an essential part of the experience of all intending doctors. Accordingly, one session a week throughout the year is devoted to the community aspects of that discipline (such as medicine, psychiatry, or child health) to which the students are attached at that time on the wards.

Perhaps the boldest part of the experiment is the assignment of nearly all the fourth year to the study of a single topic in depth. In this year one whole day a week is devoted to clinical work, and one half day is set aside to provide an opportunity for all the students in the year to meet together and discuss their projects and to introduce brief courses on such subjects as medical ethics, legal medicine, experimental design, and management.

Debates have also been held on motions such as 'The cancer patient has the right to be told the truth'. These activities have acquired the title of the fourth-year club.

Two course co-ordinators distribute students to the various options to be studied, the assignment depending on the student's wishes and the availability of suitable supervisors and laboratory and other facilities. In 1976 the 100 topics already studied included electron microscopy, insulin secretion, health education, medical care audit, metabolic rhythms, neoplastic histopathology, drug trials, epidemiology, wound healing, intrapartum asphyxia, patients' fears, psychotherapy, cross infection, calcium and vitamin D, biomechanics, stretch reflexes, teratogenesis, parenteral nutrition, chromosomes and drugs, lung function, immune complexes, bronchial metaplasia, sequelae of heart disease, renal malformations, diet, and anaemia.

At the end of the year the student has to justify his own conclusions by assessing the nature of the problem, and presenting his conclusions and the evidence on which they are based orally at a departmental meeting and in writing (not more than 5,000 words).

In the fifth year students are assigned in pairs to selected physicians and surgeons in the district general hospitals, where the students act as junior house officers. They live in the hospital. They take the history, examine the patient, keep the patient's records and discuss with the house officer the investigation, treatment, and disposal of the patient. Ten weeks are devoted to medicine, eight weeks to surgery, five to each of obstetrics and gynaecology, psychiatry, and paediatrics, and two weeks to general practice. Five weeks are allocated to an elective, usually devoted to a specialty of which the student has seen little, such as anaesthetics, neurology or neurosurgery, or orthopaedics. At the end of each attachment, the student is assessed on his notes, and on a case presentation, by his local teacher and a member of the Southampton University staff.

Judgement as to the student's attainments is made on formal examinations (Primary, Intermediary, and Final) and aided by internal assessment.

The Primary examination at the end of the first year consists of anatomy, biochemistry, and pathology. I was glad to see that in anatomy there were no artefactual questions like MCQs and true/false but straightforward questions which relate to those in real life. For the other papers MCQ questions are used and biochemistry also uses problem solving, which I commend. The periodic assessment, which is made in a variety of ways, can count up to 15 marks to the 50 necessary for a pass, but the marks for periodic assessment cannot be subtracted from those of the examination.

In March of the second year the student sits the Intermediate examination on man, medicine, and society, psychology and epidemiology. I liked the papers set in this examination (Part I of Intermediate).

Part II of the Intermediate is a mammoth examination on the systems courses, including anatomy, physiology, pharmacology, pathology and elementary medicine, and surgery. It consists of an MCQ (which is no better and no worse than its kind) which counts 30 marks, two essays counting 15 marks each, a problem solving paper counting 15 marks, and a viva counting 10 marks. One essay paper section is on pharmacology and one on biochemistry.

Internal assessment may again add 15 marks to those out of 100 gained in the formal examinations towards the pass mark of 50. Although the student will have completed some 40 weeks of clinical attachments the clinical knowledge required for the examination is limited to the understanding of pathogenesis and of disordered functions. The students are assessed on their clinical attachments in the third and fourth years, but together with the thesis written in the fourth year these do not contribute towards examination results. The thesis, however, is taken into account for the award of honours.

The final examination in June of the fifth year consists of:

1. MCQ paper of two hours' duration.

2. Two written papers each of four sections and each lasting three hours.

3. Two long cases, one medical and one surgical, including the presentation of a written case report on each.

4. A series of short cases from any discipline.

5. A 20-minute viva on clinical emergencies.

The external examiners and the GMC visitors expressed themselves as pleased with the quality of the students and their clinical competence.

The Dean comments on his 'disappointment at the prominence of the formal lecture. Of 1,320 hours' formal teaching time in the first two years about 50 per cent is devoted to lectures. While lectures have a place in transferring information, several studies have shown that they are less effective in stimulating thought or changing attitudes than projects and tutorials with active participation by the student.'

From the Science Masters' Association Report

In the construction of the syllabus we have tried to include what is both teachable and worthwhile, irrespective of its suitability or otherwise for examinations. While it is true that many of the qualities of mind which we believe our pupils may acquire from the liberal courses we have planned are beyond the scope of examinations to assess, we realize the necessity for and the powerful influence exerted by examinations. In the previous Report, very specific and, we think, very wise recommendations were made for examining in General Science. By now, however, most examining boards have adopted techniques very much in the spirit of that Report and we feel that there is no longer any need to enter into such detail. For the new General Certificate of Education we anticipate that the examination in General Science will play an increasingly important part at the 'Ordinary' level.

We emphasize that the best kind of teaching is always little influenced by the examination and we deprecate in the examination anything which would limit the freedom of the teacher to experiment or to follow, from time to time, what may appear to be profitable digressions from the syllabus. There is much more in the business of educating than the imparting of knowledge in a form readily reproducible in examinations. It is one of the dangers of any system of examinations that we may come to value only what we can test, and this peril should be ever present in the minds of both teacher and examiner.

Our predecessors laid great stress on the desirability of supplementing the written examination with further use of teachers' estimates in order to give due weight to those 'by-products' of our teaching, those 'many important qualities which cannot be valued adequately' by written tests. While we are very much in sympathy with this point of view, we realize the difficulty of standardizing such estimates. We have felt bound, therefore, to content ourselves at present with the above insistence on the limitations of written examinations, though we should welcome more research into the wider use of such estimates.

It is, of course, recognized that external examinations can exert a beneficial influence upon schools by demanding that the teaching shall not deviate too far from certain desirable paths, and in this connection we quote from the previous report:

The written tests should be compiled to attain the following objectives:

1. All the children should know thoroughly a limited range of facts and principles of fundamental importance;

2. All the courses taken in schools should cover parts of the three main sciences at least (and preferably parts of others as well);

3. This wide field should be combined with limited specialization in certain directions, i.e. teachers of science should be able to direct their attention towards topics specially relevant to the environment of their school or to their own special interests and abilities (local specialization).

One of the problems with which examiners of General Science have been faced, and one of the causes of dissatisfaction among teachers, who have prepared pupils for some of these examinations, has been that the breadth of the syllabus to be tested has made adequate sampling of its parts difficult in one examination. We are of the opinion that it is not desirable to attempt to assess the results of some five years' work over so broad a field as even our basic syllabus in a single paper. At least two papers at the 'Ordinary' level should be set. One paper should consist of a wide range of the now familiar 'New-Type' short answer questions designed to secure objectives (1) and (2) above. Another paper should consist of questions requiring essay-type answers designed to estimate certain aspects of scientific knowledge to which we attribute importance, such as the ability to marshal the points of an argument in orderly sequence or to write down clear instructions for the performance of an experiment. It should be remembered that an important part of the training we try to give to our pupils lies in the ability to express themselves with clarity in English and in this type of question candidates who have not acquired this skill are automatically penalized. It is probably inadvisable for questions of these two types, designed to test different qualities, to be incorporated in the same paper, since candidates are then tempted to answer the essay-type questions with the brevity which is encouraged in the short-answer questions. In examinations concerned with the Extended Syllabus no different principles are involved and further questions of both types are desirable.

We now give with slight modifications a list, taken from the previous Report, of the specific features with which we consider the teaching and examining of General Science to be concerned. In each case is added a question connected with that specific factor.

I. *Acquisition of Scientific Information and Knowledge.*

(i) Knowledge of empirical facts.
e.g. Name two gases which are denser than air.

(ii) Power of reproducing verbally laws or principles.
e.g. State Boyle's Law.

(iii) Knowledge of technical terms, or of words used in science.
e.g. Explain the meaning of 'latent heat'.

(iv) Ability to identify forms, structures, processes and to state their functions.
e.g. A labelled diagram of a flower is given. The candidates are asked to name the parts and to state their function.

(v) Power of explaining verbally the meaning of a law or a principle.
e.g. What is meant by Conservation of Energy? Show how this conflicts with the idea of Perpetual Motion.

II. *Development of Scientific Modes of Thought.*

(i) Ability to use scientific knowledge to explain facts of ordinary life—unification of experiences, i.e. from facts to principles.
e.g. Explain (*a*) the occurrence of the blue flame that often appears over a coal fire and (*b*) why soap forms a curdy precipitate with hard water.

(ii) Enlargement of experience by recognizing in ordinary life instances of the operation of natural laws, i.e. from principles to facts.

e.g. Describe three experiments or observations which show that thermal radiation obeys the same laws as light.

(iii) Capacity to distinguish between facts and hypotheses.

e.g. Read the following passage. Then write down:
(a) which of the statements are facts, (b) which are verifiable generalizations and (c) which are mere statements of opinion.

(iv) Isolation of relevant facts from a complex situation.

e.g. A fairly complicated experiment is described and the candidates are asked to point out which of the facts mentioned would be relevant to the solution of the problem considered.

(v) Ability to plan experiments and to test statements.

e.g. (a) How can one find out that a certain muscle in a frog's leg is an extensor and not a flexor? (b) Devise experiments to test the following statement: 'Saccharine is 500 times sweeter than sugar.'

(vi) Ability to apply generalizations to new problems.

e.g. Two identical cubes of wood are sterilized and placed in separate moist chambers. Block A is kept sterile. Block B is inoculated with a fungus, which grows and thrives in the wood. How will the dry weight of these blocks probably compare at the end of three months? Why?

(vii) Ability to draw reasonable generalizations from experimental data.

e.g. Nine hundred seeds of a certain plant were divided into nine groups of 100 seeds each. Each group of 100 seeds was placed in a germinator; they were all kept in the dark under the same conditions. But each germinator was kept at a different temperature. The following data were obtained:

Temperature, ° C.	6	8	11	13	18	25	30	35	39
Number of seeds which germinated	0	0	0	0	16	50	84	30	0

What generalizations could you draw from this experiment?

(viii) Ability to recognize problems which lend themselves to scientific treatment; and the contrary.

    e.g. Which of the following statements could be investigated experimentally and in what way?

    (*a*) Rain before seven, fine before eleven.

    (*b*) A hot-water bottle airs a bed.

    (*c*) Virtue is its own reward.

III. *Application of Scientific Knowledge to Socially Desirable Ends.*

Ability to recognize situations or unsolved problems in which scientific knowledge could usefully be employed.

e.g. (*a*) A woman planted some flower-seeds beside her house. The plants did not grow very well. The woman next door planted seeds of the same kind of flower. These plants grew very well. (*b*) A farmer had a flock of chickens. He noticed that on some days he would get many eggs and on other days he would get very few eggs. What kind of information would you need before you could explain these differences?

IV. *Practical Powers or Skills.*

Scientific knowledge involves power to use and to handle as well as power to 'talk about things'. Such skills cannot well be tested by written examinations. The candidates would have to be placed in specific situations calling for use of specific skills. The following factors can easily be distinguished.

   (i) Development of manual skill and dexterity.

   (ii) Ability to handle scientific material and apparatus (i.e. skill in laboratory technique).

   (iii) Development of ideals of careful, neat, and accurate work.

   (iv) Ability to apply scientific knowledge to solve the practical problems of everyday life.

   (v) Ability to devise experiments and to carry them through.

The material of Section IV cannot easily be tested by written examinations, but here school records might give valuable information.

When we come to consider papers at the 'Ordinary' level for more mature candidates who are probably doing advanced work in subjects other than science, it is clear that different considerations are involved. As each school may emphasize different aspects of the syllabus, the knowledge of candidates will vary widely. In any case, the testing of mere factual knowledge is relatively unimportant in this context. What the examiners will be required to elicit is evidence that the candidate has acquired some appreciation of the contribution of science to general culture, some knowledge of its methods and of its impact on society. This will mean that objective tests will probably be inappropriate and that experiments will doubtless be made with papers consisting of a liberal choice of questions of the essay type.

APPENDIX V

Surgery paper from Oxford University, June 1965

SECOND EXAMINATION FOR THE DEGREE OF BACHELOR OF MEDICINE

PRINCIPLES AND PRACTICE OF SURGERY

SECTION I

Write an essay on one of the following subjects. Candidates should devote about 1½ hours of their time to this. Due note will be taken of the form of presentation and style, as well as of the matter.

1. Surgery and ethics.

2. The problems of geriatric surgery.

3. The importance of the development of Accident Departments.

4. The importance of the collaboration of surgeon and physician in the interests of the patient.

5. Conditions mimicking carcinoma of the breast.

SECTION II

All the questions should be answered. These questions are designed to test the candidate's factual knowledge and a tabular form of answer is appropriate.

1. Enumerate the special points in the examination of a goitre.

2. In what types of fracture is some method of internal fixation the established form of treatment and why?

3. Enumerate the main causes of intra-abdominal haemorrhage.

4. In what conditions may the usual contour of the shoulder be modified?

5. What is meant by the term 'fistula in ano' and how is this condition produced?

6. What is usually the first evidence of:
   (a) sarcoma of bone;
   (b) acute intestinal obstruction;
   (c) carcinoma of oesophagus;
   (d) tuberculous kidney;
   (e) polyposis coil;
   (f) hypertrophic pyloric stenosis of infancy;
   (g) acute osteomyelitis.

7. Describe the signs and symptoms of perforated duodenal ulcer.

References

1. *Lancet* (1962), **i**, 361; *Br. med. J.* (1962), **1**, 466.
2. McLachlan, G. (ed.) (1974). *The Way Ahead in Postgraduate Medical Education* (Oxford University Press for the Nuffield Provincial Hospitals Trust).
3. *Basic Medical Education in the British Isles.* The Report of the General Medical Council Survey (1977) (Oxford University Press for the Nuffield Provincial Hospitals Trust).
4. *Report of the Interdepartmental Committee on Medical Schools* (Goodenough Report) (London: HMSO, 1944).
5. Royal Commission on Medical Education (1968). *Report 1965–68* (Todd Report), Cmnd. 3569. (London: HMSO).
6. *Universities Central Council on Admissions Clearing Statistics for 1977.*
7. Cambridge University Appointments Board (1945). *Report on University Education and Business.*
8. The National Health Service (Vocational Training) Act, 1976.
9. General Medical Council. *Annual Report for 1975.*
10. General Medical Council. *Recommendations as to Basic Medical Education, 1967.*
11. *Report of the Committee of Inquiry into the Regulation of the Medical Profession* (Merrison Report), Cmnd. 6018 (London: HMSO, 1975).
12. Churchill, W. S. (1929). Address to Bristol University.
13. Pickering, G. W. (1967). *The Challenge to Education* (London: C. A. Watts).
14. Council for Postgraduate Medical Education in England and Wales. *Report for 1971 to 1975.*
15. Medical Act, 1953.
16. *Interim Report on the Future Provision of Medical and Allied Services* (Dawson Report), Cmnd. 693 (London: HMSO, 1920).
17. Plutarch, *de Audiendo* (Loeb Classical Library: Plutarch, *Moralia*, vol. i, 256).
18. Sayers, Dorothy L. (1947–8). 'The lost tools of learning', *Hibbert Journal*, **46**, 1.
19. *Postgraduate Medical Education and the Specialties (with Special Reference to the Problem in London)* (London: HMSO, 1962).

20. *Report of the Royal Commission on University Education in London* (Haldane Report), Cmnd. 6717 (London: HMSO, 1913).
21. CRUIKSHANK, J. K., BARRETT, P. W., MCBESAG, F., WATER-HOUSE, N. and GOLDMAN, L. H. (1975). *Br. med. J.* **4**, 265.
22. SPENCE, J. C. Personal communication.
23. HALDANE, LORD (1974). In Ashby, Eric, and Anderson, Mary, *Portrait of Haldane* (London: Macmillan).
24. *Science Masters' Association Report on the Teaching of General Science* (London: John Murray, 1974).
25. ANDERSON, JOHN (1976). *The Multiple Choice Question in Medicine* (Tunbridge Wells: Pitman Medical Press).
26. FLEMING, P. R., SANDERSON, P. H., STOKES, J. F., and WALTON, H. J. (1976). *Examinations in Medicine* (Edinburgh: Churchill–Livingstone).
27. ALLAN, R. and DYKES, P. (1976). 'A study of the factors influencing mortality rates from gastrointestinal haemorrhage', *Q. Jl Med.* N.S. **45**, 335.
28. BULL, G. M. (1956). 'An examination of the final examination', *Lancet*, **ii**, 368.
29. PICKERING, G. W. (1959). 'A study of medical education in Great Britain', *J. med. Educ.* **34**, 1139.
30. ROYAL COLLEGE OF PHYSICIANS OF LONDON (1944). *Report on Medical Education*.